DID YOU KNOW THIS IMPORTANT SEX INFORMATION:

"DID YOU KNOW that people who have no feeling at all below the waist — people with spinal cord injuries, for example — can still have orgasms?

DID YOU KNOW that even if you didn't "go all the way," "just did" oral sex / cunnilingus that...

...when fresh semen is deposited on the vulva lips, even when NOT directly placed INTO the vagina, semen can still get her pregnant.

DID YOU KNOW:

That, of a survey of 1102 women, a full 11%, that's 121 women, had NEVER had an orgasm, while having conventional penis in vagina sex. But...

81% of all women REGULARLY **ACHIEVE ORGASMS FROM CUNNILINGUS** (kun'-nih-lin'-gus).

SEX GAMES FOR COUPLED ADULTS:

If something feels good, to her, or you ask her directly, she can say "Yes," or "Hot." Or purr out a, "Spicy."

"M-yes. No. Cold. Oh, yes. **Hottest**."

Or "Green Light. Green. Yel-low Light. M-Green—. Oh. Green. Ugh. Red Light."

SEXY FICTION EXCERPTS:

"Don't stop. Resume. Please?"

He didn't speak only touched her, kissed her. Everywhere. Where she had and where she had never been kissed before.

Her lips. Her face. Her neck. Her arms. Her hands. Her shoulders. Her breasts. And, oh, her breasts and belly and ... below.

Oh, below, she moaned in her mind, trying not to say such a thing aloud.

She wantonly opened her legs wide to him, at his gentle coaxing, as he moved to lie between her trembling thighs.

She wasn't certain what he might—.

"Oh!"

—erotic novel work in progress "Annamarie Makes a Match" by Neale Sourna

Have her fall completely in love with THE WAY <u>YOU</u> MAKE LOVE to her.

She'll NEVER say, "No," again.

Neale Sourna's SEXsinger:
CUNNILINGUS

How to Give Head (Oral Sex and Eating Pussy), **for Giving Women Orgasms of Cuntlicious Joy! Info and Sex Games!**

By Neale Sourna

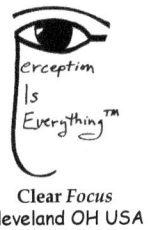

Clear *Focus*
Cleveland OH USA

Copyright © 2011 by Neale Sourna

All rights reserved. No part of this ebook may be reproduced or transmitted in any form or by any means, electronic, mechanical, magnetic, and photographic; including photocopying, recording or by any information storage and retrieval system, without prior written permission of the publisher. No patent liability is assumed with respect to the use of the information contained herein.

Although every precaution has been taken in the preparation of this book, the publisher and author assume no responsibility for any errors or omissions or apparent misinterpretations by this author, editor, or publisher, occurring between the original source materials or this interpretation.

Neither is any liability assumed for damages resulting from use of the information contained herein.

This ebook is licensed to the original purchaser only. Duplication or distribution to any other person via email, PC disk, digital file, network (wired or wifi), synch, printout, or any other means is a violation of international copyright law and subjects the violator to fines and/or imprisonment.

This notice overrides the permissions given by any software or hardware used in the production of this work, which are erroneous. This ebook cannot be lent or given to others, except by the legal permissions stipulated by the publisher at the time of licensing.

Parts of this work are works of fiction. Names, characters, places, incidents, and their juxtapositions are the product of the authors' imagination, or are used fictitiously. All informational research, unless marked as directly quoted, has been paraphrased or wholly rewritten. Any resemblance to actual specific events, locales or specific persons, living or dead, is entirely coincidental.

ISBN 978-1-938903-04-5 Print 6.14" x 9.21"

Copyrighted photos by Milzo (luscious oyster) and Zuki (lovely music) at iStockPhoto.com

Published by

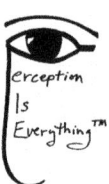

Clear *Focus*

PIE: P*erception* I*s* E*verything*™
Clear *Focus*
12600 Rockside RD Box 192
Cleveland OH 44125 USA

www.PIE-PerceptionIsEverything.com
www.PIE.Percept.com
www.Neale-Sourna.com

Librarians—nonfiction:

1. Sexuality
2. Women—Sexual behavior
3. Marriage
4. Relationships—self-improvement
5. People with disabilities—Sexual behavior

Published in the United States of America.
Printed in US, the United Kingdom, or Australia
Not for sale or republication without written permission from
PIE: Perception Is Everything/Neale Sourna

Also by Neale Sourna

Hobble
[An Adult Novel]

Steve's Monkey's Paw & MORE
[Adult Short Stories and excerpts]

North Coast Academies' Diary, Volumes 1-3
[Adult Short Stories, Fetish]

"This is Dedicated..."

"This is dedicated to the one (you) love," as the 1960s song says. And, dedicated to the one I love.

And to you, who **need** this and to you, who **want** this, may it serve you well, not steer you wrong in error, and help you find and encourage great happiness **wherever you plant your loving kisses.**

Table of Contents

DID YOU KNOW: . . . . A
Copyright © 2011 by Neale Sourna . . . . D
    Also by Neale Sourna . . . . E
    "This is Dedicated…" . . . . F
Author Statement I
    ALL ARE WELCOME HERE. I
    And what does author Neale Sourna know about it? I
    How many of us actually learned sex from a sex professional? II
    Back to "talented, dedicated amateurs" versus "paid professionals." II

Why music? III
Because, DID YOU KNOW: V
    The complete lack of knowing what to do. V
    My friends, "Ignorance is [not] Bliss." VI
  PS: Don't be tense. VII
  PPS: Challenge each other with a *Game* of *Lie and Tell*: VII
Why "Singer," "Singing," and "Sing"? VIII
    Music taught and still teaches me: VIII
    Music taught me, and still does; that… VIII

Singing is easy. IX

Why THAT Word, "Cunt"? IX
  PS: cunt XI
    And, Finally, Why the Fiction Excerpts? XI
    Author's Acknowledgements XII
  Remember: Knowledge is *powerful* XII

Neale Sourna's SEX*Singer*: CUNNILINGUS 1
Introduction. 1
    "I pulled up a chair, pushed up her skirt, and…" 2

WARNING: "Just Foreplay" 2

Best Sex EVER! For Her, With You. 2

YOUR MOST IMPORTANT SKILL: Communication. 3

    "Don't look at me!" 3

Game: Guide. 4

Game: Guide Communication Practice. 5

Game: "Silence" Game. 6

"Both of You—ALWAYS Be Positive." 6

    If you must, if she's really just not listening to you, show her these next few paragraphs: 7

    When is it over? "Since I Became Paralyzed...." 8

Research Stuff: How Her Equipment Works. 8

    Wet. 9

    Scent. 9

Hold the Fish: Vulvas Can Smell or Taste Unpleasant, Because: 9

"Taste Yourself." 10

Cunnilingus: Definition. 11

"Wait! What's Her Clitoris, and Where the Hell is It?" 11

    Cunt/Vulva Image 11

    The clitoris' ONLY job is to stimulate sexual pleasure within her. 12

    Basic Skills and Stats. 12

    "Her clitoris can be too sensitive to touch...." 13

    "Oral sex gets around issues of..." 14

Your Basic Oral Tools. 14

    Cunnilingual Movements. 15

    Education, Partners, and Restrictions. 15

    Pregnancy. 16

    "I dove. I actually dove in and licked Alice's juicy..." 17

CULTURAL, SPIRITUAL, and RELIGIOUS SIGNIFICANCE; and a BIT of LEGAL HISTORY. 17

    "Worldwide Cultural Attitudes." 18

    "Desire and Self-Esteem." 19

    "Cultural Legalities." 19

Religious Culture: Chinese Spiritual Taoism. 20
"The Great Medicine of the Three Mountain Peaks..." 20
"The practice (of cunnilingus)... 20
  Culture Philosophy: Indian Tantra. 21
  "Songs of Solomon." 21
"If Dara wished to allow the princess to touch her,...." 22

THE ICKY MEDICAL STUFF. 23
"Ew!" Yucky Stuff: STD, HPV, and Alleged Oral Cancer Risk. 23
  Personal STD control. 23
  "And, just so you know:" 24
  Oral Sex STD Prevention. 24

Warning: Dental Dam and Condom Protection. 25
  Popular Culture and Slang. 25
"Frank and Louisa are too busy to notice what we...." 25

MASTERING SexSinging BASIC ARTISTIC SKILLS. 26
Learning to Play—Your Way. 27
A Bit More on Women's Social History. 27
  "Dirty Girl"—character Baby Stewie, TV's "Family Guy." 28
  "He stared between my legs, as he slid..." 29

HELPING HER RELAX and PREPARE. 29
  "Prolonged Foreplay/Diddling. Or Fun, Creative Stuff!" 29
  "Kiss Her. Long. And Deep." 29
  "Be Kind, Unwind." 30
  Retooling Your Senses. With Her Stuff. (nonfetish) 31

Game: Your Sensitivity to Sensuality. 31
  Game: "Sensitive Sensuality, for Two." With Her Stuff. (still nonfetish) 32
  Game Interruptus: Weekend Scents. 33
  Two Hours. 34
  More Cleanliness Issues. 35
  Misc. on Pubic Hair; "To Be or Not to Be"—from William Shakespeare's "Hamlet" . .

.... 36
    You Massage Her, Sensually. 36
    "Feed me your cunt." 37

IN A HURRY? DON'T BE, OKAY, START HERE THEN. 37
    Yes, Make Your Mouth and Tongue Wet and Slippery. 38
    Don't Bash and Butt Your Hard Face into Her! 39
    When She Reacts Well to Your Action. Repeat It. 40
    When She's More Warmed Up. 41
    "Get Up and Do It, Again. Amen."—lyrics, Jackson Browne's "The Pretender" 43
    "I wiggled…" 43

NOW, BACK TO YOUR DELICIOUS MAIN COURSE 43
RE-WARNING: Don't plan it the same…. 43
Back to School, for Your "ABCs"! 44
    Game: A-B-C Sex. 44
    Sex, Sexual, Loving, Creativity. 44
Women's Advice: " 'Alphabet Letters' is Absurd." 45
    Clitoris Circling. 46
    Clitoris Sucking. 46
Warning: Highly aroused. 47
Women's Advice: "Stop Heading Down on Her…" 47
    Oyster Practice. 49
   "Dara sighed, which encouraged Tor, as he…" 49

BONUS GAMES. 50
    Game: Hornblower. 50
    Game: Red Light, Green Light. 51
    Game: Feather Your Nest. 51

POSITION(S). GET A MOVE ON. 51
    "69" [Tell the Kids, "It's the Year the Mets Won Their First World Series!"] 51
    Backward. More 69, Kind of. 52

Doggy, or, as I prefer, "Doggy-Doggy." 53
Facesitter. 53
Doggy Sit ["I think I just made this one up!"] 54
"Knees Up, Honey." 54
Legs Flat. 54
Knees, Fluid Movements, and Agony. 54
"Then his touch,…" 55

The ONLY Sex for Some. 56

MORE on COMFY POSITIONS. Yes, MORE. 56
FGM Diagram 1: 58
WARNING: Don't break rhythm. 58
"I know, I could've just taken her, I…" 59

MORE Warnings and Advice. 59
Women's Forum Advice: Again. "DO NOT Immediately Dive for Her Clitoris… 59
Women's Forum Advice: "Take Your Leisurely and Loving Time." 60
Reminder: "Be Extremely Gentle." 60
"This Pleasure's for Her; Watch, Listen, and Hear Her." 61
Insert Here. Maybe. 61
"Leith's cunt was fresh and slick, as…" 62

Male Advice 63
Paraplegic Man's Advice. 63
Paraplegic Woman's Advice: "Braingasms." 63

Lesbian Advice 64
Lesbian Forum Advice: "Put Your Nose to Her." 64
Men's Forum Advice: Warning on Fingering. 65

[Editor's Note: 65
"Orgasm: After Injury (*Physical, Emotional, or Spiritual*)." 66

More Forum Advice 66
Women's Advice: "Any oral is great oral." NO. It's Not. 66
Women's Advice: "Listen! Take notice!" 67
Women's Advice: Communicate. Ask for "Tips." 68
Game: Her Slave. 68

Game: "Sweet Nothings" and "Puppet." 69

"Ladies of the English Harem" 70

SexSinger BONUS: Add Fingersex. **71**

No "Performance." No "Task." More Training Your Senses. 72

"I *loved* him touching me. He..." 73

BEST OF BOTH—MULTITASKING: Clit AND G-spot! **73**

Putting Your Finger(s) In. 73

WARNING 1: Nails. *74*

WARNING 2: No wet spot. *74*

Squirming and Breathing Heavily. Her, Not You! 76

"Ejaculation. The Joy of 'Squirting'." 77

"I Have to Pee." 78

WARNING: Forbidden Pleasure. *78*

ANOTHER BONUS: Female Ejaculation. **78**

WARNING: Salt. *79*

Warning: Doctor's office. *79*

Focused Awareness. 80

"Go Forth, and Influence Women." **81**

Endnotes i

Author Statement

Sex, like singing or dancing, should be **enjoyable**, a **fantastic experience** of movement and intimacy, for both body and soul, and when it's not, then we're doing something wrong; whether it's oral sex, or all the other fun sexual intercourses with our loving partners.

Or, we're doing the **right** things with the **wrong** sexual love partners.

But a great deal of any wrongness can be corrected with the right information applied in the correct manner.

Sex is a skill, just like writing or singing, and can be easily improved, and sometimes made awe-inspiring.

Think about it.

You write better now, than when you were a child, don't you?

You write better alphabet letters, longer and better words, and more deep and interest content, than when you were five. And some of us can write in more than one language, even in Klingonese.

Not, everyone can do that, but **everyone can improve.**

So, THIS is something YOU CAN DO; you can IMPROVE and HAVE A TON OF FUN, by doing, and sharing.

All you need be is open and brave and willing to apply your entirely new **(for you beginners)** or your newly revamped **(for those of you more advanced in lovemaking)** skills you'll learn from this book.

ALL ARE WELCOME HERE.

ALL ARE ENCOURAGED, to **explore within these useful pages**.

Just be you.

You don't have to be red carpet movie gorgeous, smooth of silver tongued speech, or even "300" Spartan perfect warrior strong, or "The Watchmen's Dr. Manhattan"-comic book and CGI all blue male perfection, or even Olympian physically fit, in order to become a Master SexSinger, of any sex.

And neither is perfect pitch required, even you, who are tone deaf, may apply, because it's not always the tune itself, nor that it's played perfectly each and every time.

Sometimes the vibrations alone can do the trick, and bring incredible success.

* * * *

And what does author Neale Sourna know about it?

First, I'm NOT a professionally licensed medical or sexual practitioner, not in the least. Because the stuff that goes on between people would make me cry and squirm and be far too messy for me.

Okay, I'm a total pussy, under that kind of pressure.

Or would that be a total cunny?

And why is being "a pussy" an insult, hm? Think about that awhile, it's a culture thing.

But, then again, some of the most useful stuff has come from talented, dedicated amateurs and people just completely in love with the subject at hand.

Don't you have a friend who knows more about a sport or subject than the broadcast experts?

Personally, I think sex is **fascinating**, and so are **people in love**, and **in lust**. And/or both.

I mean, really:

How many of us actually learned sex from a sex professional?

Most of us, and our parents, too, learned sexual "health"—**lots of scary pictures of syphilis we HAD to look at**—from a gym teacher doing double duty in health class; or from some amateur lover a little farther ahead in the game, or more willing to experiment.

Most of us definitely didn't have a professional whore or pimp or sex therapist in that health class. And it definitely wasn't called sex class, at all.

I am, however, a professional writer in the sex and relations field, if getting paid counts.

I believe that help should be more interesting than obvious, which is why I don't usually do nonfiction. But all love and lovemaking situations are a bit in the fiction field, though, aren't they?

Back to "talented, dedicated amateurs" versus "paid professionals."

Olympians and people you know, who can sing and dance wonderfully, may never have had full training or "school learnin' " or have been given a record deal, or a certificate for their wall that states that they are a "Sex Expert."

Sometimes, they're much more interesting than those who have studied "by the book" or were sanctioned by some outside sanctioning group; but now have **nothing new or fresh to add**.

So, I'm a thinking AND feeling writer, and a professional, yes, I actually gets paid for this; sex writer in the field of creative sex writing **(fiction and nonfiction)**, which means I observe, research, analyze, and translate what I comprehend of culture, personality, and interpersonal relationships through the loving filter of my own—**precious to me**—body and knowledge and feelings.

If I feel it, that warm, "naughty" feeling, don't you think or feel or whatever it is that you do, that a few 6 or 7 million other people, or at least a nice portion of them, might just feel something similar?

That's connection, my friend. We don't have to talk person to person about it; we KNOW it's there, the human connection.

Heart to page to heart.

I then I take the feelings and thoughts and research and culture, etcetera and combine it together in a new way and put it all into more easily understood way, that's conversational and fun, and that has strong personal feeling and personal meaning for you, Happy Reader and Sexual Explorer, just like making love does.

Exactly like making love. Same parts, same number of combinations, but different results, because we're all different, in wonderful ways.

Writing to me is a form of lovemaking, especially in creative fiction; so, I guess, I love you. I hope you love me, too.

Why music?

I've a background in music history, composition, advanced harmony, and in vocal singing and playing an instrument—**piano, recorder, clarinet, French Horn**—which include high skill in articulate lips, flexible tonguing, fingering, and breath.

And if you think the title and the subject of this book are scandalous, then you should see the things musicians do with their mouthpieces!

Especially in marching band, and it's freezing cold in the American Midwest!

Oh, yes, and I believe in utter egoless joy and delicious pleasure, much like we experienced as children, before we were told to "grow up" and be frozen, self-conscious, "mature" people, afraid that any thing sexual is "dirty," "not of true interest," or "shouldn't be fun," because so many of us experience so little joy, and so rarely.

That changes NOW!

Because, THE BEST WAY TO HAVE JOY is to GIVE JOY.

So, this is Educated Opinion's Advice, culled from the Actual Experience of others and self, and from Creative Imagination, hand sculpted into a TANGIBLY USABLE FORM for YOUR Sexual EDUCATION, YOUR Oral FUN, and YOUR Sexual, Oral PLEASURE.

Well, actually, for HER PLEASURE **and** your delicious pleasure, in pleasing her. Because causing pleasure and joy in another, especially in someone you love, is a great orgasmic and often ecstatic feeling of its own.

And worth all the more to me, and to you, than all that bull of what is often passed off as sexual pleasure, but isn't. You've cried enough tears to know that it isn't.

Or she has.

If you still think I'm not qualified, that's your right; but, remember, how many times have you asked your well-schooled doctor or professor or other licensed professional an important question, that was HIGHLY IMPORTANT TO YOU, and they never actually answered, to your SATISFACTION, or just clearly LEFT YOU HANGING, EXPOSED and UNFULFILLED, because they too aren't expert in everything and can be miseducated, too.

Or just are still afraid, this late in the game, to be open and brave about pleasure, especially sexual pleasure.

And, let's face it, how many of these ineffective advisors of yours actually ever studied Basic Human Bodily Pleasure, Intermediate Human Bodily Pleasures, let alone Advanced Human Bodily Pleasures, Graduate Studies Level.

None?

And, just like you, these "experts" are often unfulfilled, too, sexually.

But would they ever tell you?

Or do they, perhaps, say, "That's just the way it is"?

It's not. It's "just the way it was."

I mean really DO YOUR EXPERTS, who you depend on for useful, truthful sexual information, LOOK HAPPY and RELAXED, to you, and like they're sexually sated?

I doubt it.

Or they'd be fixing it for you, too; overjoyed to share the recipes, techniques, and method melodies that have put a smile on their faces, a song deep in their hearts and throats.

Or selling their technique on talk TV!

Now, that would be fun, probably, but that's clearly NOT MY GOAL, or I'd change my title to something more politically correct, more media friendly.

For this, I'm not the media's friend, I'm yours.

Because I LOVE sex and love and I want to share this with you.

* * * *

And, as bold as I sound, and am, I'm also just as shy about a lot of this as you or your special her is. That's why we pass folded, secret notes in class, to say what we can't say aloud, to pass on our joy and hope it's well-received.

This is my love note on tongue loving to you in the world, in hopes a few more or a million or billion more women, and their loving partners, will HAVE and SHARE **GREAT JOY**.

Because happy women MAKE the world happy!

So, lovey, unwrap the package, it's Christmas EVERY NIGHT, and DAY.

And we can do this, YOU CAN DO THIS.

Hey. We pump our own gas, we load our own software. We can figure out together a little friendly, personal yet universal sense about what to do during a little one on one tasty playtime alone together.

* * * *

Okay, for the hardcore doubters, **still** wondering, "What the hell does Neale Sourna really know about sex?"

Besides having a fairly extensive private library about it.

Besides being a professional sex writer, editor, and publisher.

Well, I've also co-ghostwritten and edited a male masturbation book and successfully written for several relationship, romance, and sex sites online; through my writing company www.Writing-Naked.com.

But, enough about me, because **this is all about you AND her.**

SexSinger: Cunnilingus

* * * *

Because, DID YOU KNOW:

That, of a survey of 1102 women, a full 11% had NEVER had an orgasm.[1] And that 46% of these women thought ALL MEN WERE SELFISH; while a high "79 percent thought only their husbands were selfish."

Ouch.

Plus, 56 % of these married women still believed the old beehive and stiletto heels time's sexual propaganda that some women, many women are frigid, intentionally and stubbornly so, which was a standard 1950s-60s Cold War way to batter a woman, whether wife or passing partner, not sexually interested or satisfied, but unknowing how to correct it.

That "real women" aren't interested in sex, "only sluts." Not realizing real, sweet and loving women were and are interested, but that the love her lover was making to her or with her was ignorant, or inadequate to the task.

It was pleasure for everyone in the room, but her. And still is.

And they wondered why she wasn't interested?

It wasn't HIS fault, it was ALL HER FAULT.

To put that on the other foot, considering that many men have a problem with their sexual function, so much so it has a cute name now, ED **[erectile dysfunction]**, how much have men LOVED being called "impotent" or "not a real man," because his sexual interest was taking a nosedive, failing to rise to the occasion, etcetera?

Not much, I'm thinking.

That same beehive culture, from which we're now descended, said that both a woman and a man, but most especially all women needed no sexual education before her wedding night, except her mother telling her on her wedding day that her new husband will do "unpleasant things to her" and that she had "to endure it."

Wow. Doesn't sound joyful ... and fun, to me, or like everyone knows all they need about sex.

Add to this widely cultural ignorance, which is still threaded throughout our culture(s):

The complete lack of knowing what to do.

Especially with her and for her, or of how her wonderful, fascinating body works in an intimate, nakedly open, and face to face sexual context.

But then, voila, on her wedding night, she's told to open wide, AFTER being screamed at about "keep your knees closed" since the second she was born a girl child and her family and world decided her best and only protection was total, obliterating ignorance.

And when has **ignorance** really ever come in handy, especially when something needs to be physically done?

---

[1] Hayden, Naura. How to Satisfy a Woman EVERY Time ... and Have Her Beg for More! New York: Bibli O'Phile Books, Inc., 2001. pp. 85-86

"Oh, gee, I smell gas; let me light this match afire to see for certain." "Oh, that looks sharp, but I won't know for certain not until I chop my hand with it."

My friends, "Ignorance is [not] Bliss."

Well, that world and attitude hasn't changed yet, not as much as one, or I, would've hoped.

Not yet.

But we—you and I—are working on it.

Right now.

Inhale a deep, cleansing and filling breath, and be thankful, that YOU CAN CHANGE YOUR PART OF THAT WORLD AND ATTITUDE.

Yes, you, because....

* * * *

THIS IS ABOUT HER **and** YOU, together; and the tantalizing anticipation, then wonderful actual feel and smell and taste of great sex, and our total submergence into **wonderful** sex shared between two **wonderful** people.

* * * *

Fortunately for you and me, various other researches, so that we can learn and improve, have shown and proved that:

81% of all women REGULARLY **ACHIEVE ORGASMS FROM CUNNILINGUS (kun'-nih-lin'-gus),**...

...compared to a mere lowly 25% of women, who get orgasms FROM traditional penile penetration.

Meaning that penis in cunt penetration stimulation alone, without additional help, like adding clitoral stimulation, DOESN'T GET HER OFF, doesn't make her cum.

You get the picture. I hope.

* * * *

Now.

Which would **you** rather have, when YOU'RE receiving sex, 81% of success or just a random, once in a while 25%?

Think $81 or, I'm good; just pay me $25, instead.

Hell no.

So, let her see how much unconditional LOVE and open GRATITUDE you have for being able to "give," to encourage her pleasures and ecstasies, and the fantastically great HONOR that is yours, that she has allowed YOU to be THE ONE to be HER PLEASURE GIVER, HER ... MASTER SEXSINGER.

Enough said.

Enjoy.

You must be thirsty and starving for oral pleasure.

I know she is.

—Neale Sourna

PS: Don't be tense.
- Take a deep breath, and let it out.
- Take another deep, full breath.
- Let go of all mental concepts, emotional anguish, and all wayward thoughts of what you *should be* and what you *should be* doing.
- Relax.
- Tickle each other.
- Tell each other a few stupid jokes.

PPS: Challenge each other with a Game of *Lie and Tell*:

Think of one sincere thing that's a lie, and one sincere thing that's a truth, but mix up which one you tell first. One of you goes first and tells one of your two brief stories. The other person goes. Then you switch back and finish. Then discuss.

What's so much fun about this? You can make them very TRUTHFUL, sincere lies, or….

As I prefer, tell REALLY HUGE TALL TALE-type LIES, because they're MORE FUN for my listener.

And the sincere truth, I keep real and fairly modest, because both of our stories, both truth and lie, tell our loving partners much about us, and puts them right with us, in the same place, in the same state of mind and heart.

Now. Go have fun.

Why "Singer," "Singing," and "Sing"?

Singing is easy; although singing well, is a little harder, but don't let that bother you; it doesn't bother many inductees to the music Grammy Awards, as many famous, professional "singers" are technically and even stylistically imperfect, so YOU can do as well as them, or better.

Singing is musical invention; whether it's simple tunes and fanciful drones or complicated harmonies that soar and fall and swoop and go intricately round and round, then distill back into a simple tune, as simple as her bright-eyed smile.

* * * *

I don't work as a singer, musician, marching band instructor, or composer of music.

And yet, I use my music everyday.

The same Sonata Allegro form that Beethoven used I use to write novels, screenplays, and short stories; and the occasional poem.

Or nonfiction books about sex and sexual fun!

Music taught and still teaches me:

- musicality;
- about being melodious and harmonious;
- finding pleasure in perfect tones and the interesting variety of intense, discordant tones and the restful pauses found between them.

Music taught me, and still does; that...

...there should be diversity, there should be ups and downs, and side to sides, louds and softs. Cross tones that are harmonious, and some that clash, some that vibrate and tickle and, some that bring you back to restful harmony, where you'll enjoy it all the more, because of your wild journey.

It's not unlike an itch which you delay scratching, and then have true ENJOYMENT when you do FINALLY "scratch that itch."

Music taught me, to make internal, complimentary changes of the master key or theme, which changes the feel of the song I sing or play out, but which keeps it familiar.

Music taught me that once you have a theme or rhythm stated, you expand and explore it, and examine it from different angles and attitudes and let it grow, until it bursts in crescendo, then you resolve it all to peace; Sonata Allegro form.

Music taught me to let go as much as I can and relax and yet focus and practice my art, at least twenty (20) minutes a day, until I find my melodies and my voice, which is when it becomes enjoyable—sex is usually easier, but doesn't always last that long.

It can and should, if it's a complete song or symphony.

And it will for you, because now YOUR ART is to find YOUR VOICE, which is YOUR SEXUAL CENTER, whether in music, or in a "writer's voice," or a "character's voice," for those writers among us.

SexSinger: Cunnilingus

We're writing and singing love here; for YOUR SONGS, in YOUR VOICE, your sexual voice that is YOU and YOURS, and NO ONE ELSE's.

It's the same as when someone says, "I knew it was you, when I heard your voice!" And they're **happy** to hear you. Because YOUR sound WAS MUSIC to **their** ears.

Singing is easy.

It's not "hard" or "difficult."

And so should sex be.

But singing does take focus. And practice. If you want to do well, and not make others cringe, and flinch at the sound of it!

You don't have to be a virtuoso with "perfect pitch," either; because even bad singers and boring singers, and just plain **weird** singers, can become famous and legendary.

You already know that music is individual—**some like African jungle drums, some like Native American handmade flute tones, some only listen to Spanish-Polish Polka**—music is for the ears, but also for the body, like a drum roll or your favorite cranked up dance music vibrating through you.

My advanced classes taught all of us classmates, **music can be visual AND emotional**.

And anyone in heartfelt love, or heartfelt lust, too, can know the fine music of the body's dance, of two bodies together, shifting from vocalizing two inner, separate, and conflicting tunes, as they shift and change, and become more open.

And then meld into ONE FINE HARMONY of combined voices, whose bodily vibrations harmonize and blend together, into beauty.

Into sexual beauty.

Why THAT Word, "Cunt"?

You're thinking, "Well, that was all poetic and stuff, but why do you have to use **that** word, the c-word? It's **soooo** vulgar."

Is it?

My truest, heart and soul-felt answer: "Why not? It's an ancient word that was not slanderous or a curse word, even less so than vagina, or vulva, but has been used as an accusatory negative, much like the word 'feminist,' as in, You're NOT a 'feminist,' ARE you?"

And let's face it one hears slang terms of women's parts more than the true titles. When was the last time you heard "vulva" spoken on broadcast TV or radio? And didn't you grow up hearing "boobs" and "tatas" more than "breasts" or "down there" more than the cumbersome and specific "female sexual organs"?

And, that's all I've got to say, there's an entire thick little book called,

"Cunt," by Inga Muscio, if you want more details on whether you want to detox off your fear of the word.

And whether it is truly an "obscene" word, or just a stupendously abused **female** word. The **ultimate** female word, as Ms. Muscio'd say; because **no man** has one.

Let's face it most people don't even really know what cunt is, or means, except they assume it's THE c-word you shouldn't say; especially when spoken of in front of mom, grandma, and other respected women.

Sometimes it's "Cocksucker" or some such other c-word, too, but you can only tell by the fumbling, cultural context, as all the kids and teens in the area put their heads together to figure it out!

Even those who study words can't seem to "get to the bottom" of exactly where the word comes from, and exactly what it means.

Personally, I put it with "bitch," which also wasn't a bad word back in ancient days, and a "son of a bitch" wasn't what you think it is. The guy partied with the ladies and then got sacrificed to death, by being ripped apart by women.

Ouch!

And the late Peter Jennings, super news U.S. anchor was the first mainstreamer I ever heard say "bitch" on nationwide US TV, about a famous woman defendant. Now, everyone says it.

Geez, when actress Lucille Ball was pregnant in the 1950s on US TV, they never mentioned the word "pregnant." Let alone vulva or vagina, because anything under the clothes, especially of female origin has to be digitized out or euphemized. Like "boobs," "bazooms," "cha-chas," and tons more nonsense words for breasts.

And why don't they digitize and hide fat men's breasts on TV? Because men's breasts are BETTER than women's? Or less obscene? Hell no.

Please, digitize those puppies, people!

And the only TV word at all, that were allowed in the not so olden days, for a woman's most private bits, was the word "womb."

Which clearly makes one think, "Oh my god, is that ALL it can be used for? Giving painful birth's NOT FUN."

And also it was forbidden to say the word "condom" on US TV far into the 1980s.

While back in the 1880s and 1780s on back a woman was supposed to feel offended, if her husband offered to wear a condom, while having sex with her, whether he had a disease like syphilis or she was on her fourteenth baby in twelve pregnancy fattening years of "marital bliss."

Why was **this** "logic" their "honorable" attitude?

Because men only wear THOSE THINGS with sex-selling, demented, and evil females called whores and prostitutes. Ah, for shame.

And quite recently, this 21st century, everyone got all queasy when actress, activist Jane Fonda said, "the c-word" in a TV interview.

Anyway, why cunt all **in your face?** Well, duh. Because this is about cunnilingus; licking cunt, you silly goose!

So, happy cunt to you and yours. We all came out of one, even you test tube types.

PS: cunt

Cunt *(older Germanic word [origin 1275-1325] — English is a Germanic language — for Neo Latinate vagina [origin 1675-1685]; but there are still some language masters arguing over the REAL origins of cunt)*, cunctipotent *(all powerful, female style)*, cunning, cunny *(nickname for cunt, think pussy, or coney for rabbit)*, kin, kinsman.

Also *cunnilinctor*[2]: A male performing oral-sex on the clitoris and vulva.

Synonyms: cunnilingist; cunnilinguist.

See also: *cunnilinctrice*[3]: A female performing oral-sex on the clitoris and vulva.

Synonyms: cunnilingist; cunnilinguist.

And, Finally, Why the Fiction Excerpts?

Why the fiction, and some nonfiction, excerpts? Because most women **love** interesting stories of character and interrelationships, some with gentle romance, some with horny explicitness.

So, to help you and give you cues on what kinds of things might be good to add to YOUR foreplay, to YOUR diddling, to whatever gets YOUR favorite her wet and ready, I've included various fiction clips, as a sampler.

Yes, most are mine, but then I don't have to worry about legal clearances or whether I got a quote EXACTLY right. Right?

I'm lazy, get over it. And, I **really** like my stuff, and want to share. There's also plenty other things your local librarian, bookstore, or internet connection can hook you up in your search for great, loving, erotic reads that suit you both.

If she likes the excerpts, read more like them to her, and let her read to you, as you two cozy together, and warm each other.

In pleasure and the pleasure of togetherness.

And the nonfiction bits may just add to your info facts mental list, and also actually add a new dimension or two of possibilities to your lovemaking.

All in all, read her some horny, sexy, delicious fiction and she'll get horny, sexy, and delicious with you.

---

2 www.sex-lexis.com/Sex-Dictionary/cunnilinctor
3 www.sex-lexis.com/Sex-Dictionary/cunnilinctrice

Author's Acknowledgements

Thanks to Wikipedia and all its fine editors **(I'm one, so I thank myself, too.)**, and also online internet world sex forums, resources, and the wonderfully educational Cleveland Public Library.

And Landmarks' Son of Citation Machine at http://citationmachine.net/.

And several really great and informative sex books I always keep close to hand.

You should too.

I also thank the teachings of Joe Vitale, Caroline Myss, Les Brown, Edgar Cayce, Lynn V. Andrews, and Carlos Castaneda for inspiration on all planes of existence.

Remember: Knowledge is *powerful*

— not just power.

Relaxation opens the heart for love to both enter and step forth, heart welcomes and translates inspiration from paradise and beyond, into livable substance and action, and all together they equal fun in bed, and in our bodies and emotions.

And, as screenwriters Chris Matheson and Ed Solomon, the fine creators, who gave birth to the wonderful "Bill and Ted" films and cartoon, will always continue to say:

"Be excellent to each other; and . . . party on, dudes!"[©4]

---

4 "Bill & Ted's Excellent Adventure" (1989 film) and "Bill & Ted's Bogus Journey" (1991 film) and "Bill & Ted's Excellent Adventures" (1990, 1992 TV cartoon series). Reference www.IMDB.com (Internet Movie DataBase).

Neale Sourna's SEXSinger: CUNNILINGUS

How to Give Head (Oral Sex and Eating Pussy), for Giving Women Orgasms of Cuntlicious Joy! Info and Games!

By Neale Sourna

Introduction.

You have a delicious dream and a warm-hearted need to please her, or more precisely to "give her pleasure," and you have the desire to be THE ONE she calls to her, and keeps close to her, when she does wants happy and warm pleasure, because NO ONE BUT YOU makes her enjoy her own body the way you do.

Perhaps, you've not been able to be this person for her, or several hers have come and gone, whether pleased or not pleased, satisfied or not satisfied, but it's left you disheartened.

Because, maybe you felt or were told that you'd failed her.

Even when you hadn't.

Or, maybe, you had.

That doesn't matter, because the statute of limitations is over on all that. Every new woman is a new start, and EVERY STEADY LADY IS A NEW WOMAN; different than she was yesterday, different than she was an hour ago.

You may "sigh" another big, disheartened "sigh" here.

Okay, now, **that's enough self pity.**

Well, frankly, IT REALLY ISN'T YOUR FAULT.

There's a LOT of misinformation and false bravado out there, falling from false lips and dated information pages, passed down and repeated from long before your parents were born.

And, no, I'm not EVEN going to swear that I, and I alone, have and know ALL THE ANSWERS, nor that I CAN TEACH YOU **EVERYTHING** YOU NEED TO KNOW ABOUT WOMEN!

"That's just crazy talk."—Nathan Petrelli, TV show "Heroes"

Well, the falsehoods and obvious misdirections and outdated moralities end here, as **we kick them to the curb** and tell them:

"I don't need you; I've found a BETTER way. More than ONE way, in fact. So, goodbye liars. Hello, my sweet honey, I'M YOUR BEST LOVER."

And, how can you possibly lose, my friend?

Her ENTIRE body is an erogenous zone, and ALL her layers of senses, emotions, and fertile mind are at YOUR disposal, and command; EVERYTHING, under YOUR CONTROL—scent, taste, touch, hearing, even spirit and daydreams, and her "Oh, yeah, I'm feelin' yah" vibe, too.

So, my friend, ENTER HERE. And smile as you do. But, watch the teeth, partner.

============================

"I pulled up a chair, pushed up her skirt, and…"

"…and the sight of her, the smell of her passed through me, like the sensuous, intimate touch of soft silk on a bare, aroused nipple.

"She lay back, luxuriously stretching out across the dinner table, confident that I'd get to all the best parts, in good time. I knew she was overdue, and so was I, when her fingers tantalizingly produced a stream of juice that flowed from the deepest valley of her sex. I dove in, tongue first, until her gyrations against my face were so rough and inviting and in desperate need of me, that I…."

—from Neale Sourna's "Hobble" *(a Year's Best Erotica Novel Award Winner)*; available now, ebook and/or print

----

WARNING: "Just Foreplay"

NEVER think of cunnilingus as "JUST FOREPLAY" and something to just get her ready before you get to the "main event." It is the main event for her, and it can be wonderful for you, too.

Don't plan it the same every time; sometimes you have a little "c" time, sometimes a little "f" time (for those of you with a penis or a penis prop or nice fingers or…).

Cunnilingus is fine of and by itself.

You may continue onto all that thrusting and writhing, or switch off on each other, or you may just hug, cuddle, and rest together. Really sleep, in relaxed trust, when sleeping together.

Best Sex EVER! For Her, With You.

Cunnilingus, for most women, is the single best way for you to intensify her orgasms and your overall experience and sexual skill ability together, as a couple, in lovemaking.

Let's rarely use the word "technique," because, sometimes, it sounds like we're doing it, making our sex fun, by boring, mindless habit, repeating and repeating the same tedious thing, over and over again.

That's not for us; because that's NOT GOOD ENOUGH FOR YOU, and especially not for HER.

What you're doing, by reading this, by absorbing this, and by putting it INTO ACTION in both your lives, isn't that, instead, YOU'RE GAINING and PERFECTING a fantastic SKILL, that will MAKE **YOU** SHINE in HER **BRIGHT EYES**.

She'll have THE BEST sex she's EVER had, with your mastery, and become HER MASTER CUNNING LINGUIST[5]!

And that is VERY good, isn't it?

Now, read on.

YOUR MOST IMPORTANT SKILL: Communication.

Remember: in sex and love, communication IS NOT a bad thing; and that IT FLOWS in both directions, between you—and that ITS POWER SHOULD BE ALLOWED TO FLOW FREELY, like it flows between magnet and iron, holding each fast to the other; eye to eye, toe to toe, kiss to kiss, heart to heart and sex to sex.

And, your **mutual** communication is **multileveled**; words, sounds and utterances, signs and expressions, touch, and more. Yes, there's more.

But, first tell her that she must give you, her lover, a boon, a gift of verbal guidance, in the same way she'd guide a blind person, whom she can't touch, but who, with her loving assistance, must learn and find his way, along a confusing and dangerous city street.

This blind person MUST receive a great deal of detailed, accurate instructions. Or be lost forever.

And for any of us who've interrupted our busy day or all too brief lunch break to help a blind person find their way to their first day of college, for instance, as I did **many** years ago; you always feel in remembrance the fine pleasure of having helped someone to successfully find their way, someone who really NEEDED YOUR ASSISTANCE, when no one else could or would do.

So, CLOSE YOUR EYES before her, and TELL HER, in your own words and way:

"I'm blind and I'm feeling lost, and am afraid that I'll never find my way alone; but, I feel that **only** you know what I need to know and **only** you are kind enough to show me, and that you are the **only** one I trust, to lead me where I cannot see my way. Will you help me, please?"

Yeah, it's a bit mushy; but, trust me, mushy's good, when you're naked and open to each other. And if you can't do a little mushy, open-hearted love play between you; then WHAT ARE YOU **DOING?**

* * * *

"Don't look at me!"

If you haven't already, close or reclose your eyes, and let **her** lead you. It's HER BODY, so she gets to control.

Closing your eyes gets you out of the driver's seat, and out of pretending

---

5 Cunning linguist from cunnilingist or cunnilinguist: A person who performs oral-sex on the female genitals. Synonyms: cunnilinctor; cunnilinctrice; cunniliguist; cunnilinguant; cunnophile . See cunnilinctor and cunnilinctrice for more synonyms.

www.sex-lexis.com/Sex-Dictionary/cunnilingist

you know where you're going, when you quite plainly don't. Ladies, stop laughing.

It also allows her not to have to make eye contact before she's warmed up to it all, and showing you her full on "O-face." **[O for orgasm]**

Also, for myself I hate making eye contact, sometimes, with people, because I'll start the cataloging, as I automatically start worrying or considering and reconsidering every look, glance, and expression in their eyes and on their face.

"Eyes are happy, but mouth isn't."

"Eyes look perplexed, mouth looks determined, and that little frowny thing, between the brows means what, right now; happy or thoughtful or...?"

So, close your eyes, and let her have her face to herself and you can concentrate on her voice and touching her.

Besides, she'll have that time to REALLY look at you and SEE, for herself, the JOY YOU FEEL, in exploring her and enjoying giving her pleasure!

* * * *

Many women still feel exceedingly uncomfortable giving sexual commands and demands; feeling, to their core, that it's unfeminine.

Yes, they know better, but **feeling** rules here.

And some, whether of the younger generations or of an older one, long tired of "the rules," know they need to be sexual instructors, of what pleases and displeases them, if they expect to get what they truly want and really need, in bed.

But, she's not a drill sergeant, my friend, unless of course she REALLY is a drill instructor, serving in the armed services, that is.

Game: Guide.

Make a fun game of her giving you her assistance in teaching and training you, and tell her that HER GUIDANCE can come in the form of **verbal** commands, **auditory** sounds, hand **gestures**, and body **movements**.

Her auditory sounds, whether words, grunts, hums, sighs, or whatever, are quite useful, especially if the woman receiving your love attentions is hesitant in any fashion, such as apparently feeling that she'd be "pushy," "unladylike," or "overbearing," by giving commands and orders to you, about her intimate pleasures.

Or she just doesn't want to **distract** herself **away** from her **full focus** in feeling all her wonderful, pleasurable sensations, **that you're making her feel**, by trying to speak actual words, phrases, or sentences.

And, don't forget the BIGGER picture.

If she knows or believes others outside your room or house or whatever area, inside or outside, that you're making love in, she may be more hesitant to verbalize.

If, however, your love nest is safely private and/or soundproofed, her vocal sounds can provide a LOT of feedback to you, if the she wants to give it.

Her "Oooing, cooing, moaning, purring, trilling, grunting, panting, shouting, screaming or ... **singing**"—I like that one and the "trilling" a lot—in a variety of volumes and speeds, in physical and emotional response to what she likes, or loves that you're doing with her, and to her, can **literally** speak volumes, between the lines, while your pleasure-giving lip and tongue servicing "plays" her, you're FAVORITE, delicate instrument, in a good way.

A great way.

An instrument playing itself is a neat novelty—player piano—but it doesn't give as much satisfaction as playing that precious instrument yourself, because each "instrument" will play and sing different tones and flavors and melodies than when another person **plays the exact same instrument**.

It's like the audible difference between Joe Walsh and Eric Clapton and BB King. Or the varying differences Sheryl Crowe, Ella Fitzgerald, and Björk. And then there's that teen next door, who's practicing to get into the marching band at university, who's a fine player, but sounds distinctly different from Herb Alpert and Louis Armstrong, in their tonguing, breaths, tones, and fingering.

Yes, you may smile at that, now.

Game: Guide Communication Practice.

If something feels good, to her, or you ask her directly, she can say "Yes," or "Hot." Or purr out a, "Spicy."

If something doesn't feel good, to her, she can say, "No" or "Cold." Or "Flat."

Just like the old children's game, "Am I getting hot?" Or the other one, "Red Light, Green Light."

But instead of, "Are you getting hot, hotter...?"

"M-yes. No. Cold. Oh, yes. **Hottest**."

Or "Green Light. Green. Yel-low Light. M-Green—. Oh. Green. Ugh. Red Light."

Get the picture?

Hear the audio track?

And feel free to find and pick your own game words. It's YOUR GAME.

Also.

Remember: in sex and love, communication IS NOT a bad thing; and that IT FLOWS in both directions, between you—and that ITS POWER SHOULD BE ALLOWED TO FLOW FREELY, like it flows between magnet and iron, holding each fast to the other; eye to eye, toe to toe, kiss to kiss, heart to heart and sex to sex.

And, your **mutual** communication is **multileveled**; words, sounds and utterances, signs and expressions, touch, and more. Yes, there's more.

Game: "Silence" Game.

Don't speak.

You can leave your eyes open for this, but DON'T SPEAK.

This should keep you both from getting stuck on words and also on the tone of the words you speak, or what the meaning of each word or phrase means, or its hidden meanings, when you or she specifically say them.

Yes, some of us think and overthink, incessantly. So....

Don't speak.

Simply, SHE MUST GIVE YOU DIRECTIONS and YOU MUST FOLLOW THEM, but you MUST communicate WITHOUT words, ONLY signs, sighs, and perhaps grunting, and that delicious trilling.

Of course, this opens all kinds of doors, if your favorite her is a psycho babe; but my nephew always says, "Psycho babes are the best." But, that's usually during "Buffy: The Vampire Slayer" DVD marathons, I've never asked if that includes real girls.

Now, back on point.

No speaking.

Charades, silent charades, if you must.

Whistles, if you can.

Well, **she** can, **your** lips and tongue are **too busy,** for whistling.

"Both of You—ALWAYS Be Positive."

Keep her relaxed, and yourself, too. How? Simple. Don't take it all so stiff and serious.

Pause and joke a little bit, in a relaxed, good-natured way.

Or tell a brief, bad "Ahhh!" kind of joke.

Or go back to that little ticklish spot on her. But, don't maker her throw up, fool. If she hurls all over your lovemaking spot, she'll probably be too embarrassed or too pissed to let you touch her again.

Just try a little tickle to relax, but not so much that it gives her stomach cramps and causes her to hurl up her last meal. Y'know, that expensive dinner you just bankrupted your account on her behalf.

Why relaxing, though?

Because, when you're **both** relaxed, the joy and pleasure rise and fill you easier than when you're tense. The tense stuff is porno joy juice for your sexual mind, but it doesn't make for the best or even good REAL sex, but, being relaxed and untense does.

Tell her she can grasp your head **(the one on your shoulders)**—"But, be careful with your nails, baby."—and guide your mouth on her, in order steer you to where she wants you to give her pleasure, next.

If she wants you to stay put, she can wrap her legs around you and hold you in place.

Or tap you on the shoulder of head, like a good, good ... mmmm....

Do know, for your information, and **gently** let her know, too, that, while many women fear that they'll chase a sex partner away, by being **too** demanding in bed, they can also definitely lose a few lovers or husbands, if she's apparently seeming to be entirely impassive and indifferent to her lover's gentle and loving efforts.

Most guys HATE that.

And, yes, as most of us know, some guys like a "dead fish," morgue girl; and some girls like being a Limp Lisa; but, that's something you'll have to workout between you.

But, generally, it's not "feminine" or "sexy," to many men, if their woman's just merely lying there, and is as inappreciative as a lifeless lump of shoe heel dirt, lying wherever it lays, and not interested in her own sexuality or pleasure, as she just lies there, unmoving and staring at the ceiling, wall, or floor, facing whatever direction you last left her in, and **enduring it all,** and "thinking of England"[6], and being less lively than a zombie wife, who'd, at least, try to eat your brains!

We're not thinking of zombies here.

We're thinking of lovers, and how they feel and taste. Yum.

The person performing cunnilingus should look, really look, deep into their partner's eyes for guidance, communicating with their eyes, when silent, and verbally, when that is the game, asking her if she likes what they're doing with her and to her.

Because the eyes lie less often about the truth within than the lips.

* * * *

If you must, if she's really just not listening to you, show her these next few paragraphs:

You, the receiving woman, should BE HONEST with your love partner.

"DON'T LIE" and "NEVER fake" your pleasure or orgasm; because YOU are teaching your lover bad habits, by making them believe that what they are doing truly gives you pleasure.

And then, soon, you'll whine and whine about NEVER being satisfied with someone YOU YOURSELF TAUGHT to misLove you.

---

6 The phrase "lie back and think of England" is an expression supposedly from the United Kingdom during the Victorian Era. Traditionally, it was advice given to a new bride, about having sexual intercourse with her husband. The phrase origins are unclear, but is normally attributed to Lady Alice Hillingdon (1857-1940), as written in her journal in 1912 (Edwardian Era): "I am happy now that George calls on my bedchamber less frequently than of old. As it is, I now endure but two calls a week, and when I hear his steps outside my door I lie down on my bed, close my eyes, open my legs and think of England."

That's not fair to him, her, or to your real pleasure.

You're legs are open, you should be open too, and be honest; because, in love and lovemaking, you truly "get what you give."

===========================

When is it over? "Since I Became Paralyzed…."

"Since I became paralyzed in both legs, I have noticed that I have varying kinds of orgasms, depending upon the situation. [*Much the same for unparalyzed women, too!*]

"For example, when I play with myself and rub my clit a certain way, my orgasms are much more intense. Sometimes my leg will go into spasm and my crotch feels tingly. But, when I am with my lover, I find that it is more difficult to have an orgasm, even if he is doing EVERYTHING right.

"I think it is because I rely on the sensation of my fingertips on my clit and lips and I am able to change how hard I press or how fast I rub, based on how my clit feels on my fingertips.

"Sometimes, this is hard to explain to a lover because I am not always able to communicate clearly when I am feeling more sexually aroused.

"Eventually, I do have an orgasm, and though they are satisfying, they are not at physically intense. I realize how it might be helpful for my lover to know what it is that I feel, when I am masturbating, so he knows what he may need to change or do differently."

In our view, too much is made of the finale of a sexual response. It's almost as if without a "proper" ending (which the experts always consider to be an orgasm) the experience somehow isn't valid. [edit] …we suggest that you give yourself permission to consider *anything* at *all* to be the proper end of a sexual experience.

— *The Ultimate Guide to Sex and Disability*[7]

[*It will end when it ends; when you part or fall asleep together, or….*]

Research Stuff: How Her Equipment Works.

Her vulva[8] should be moist because her vaginal shaft and vulval lips are constantly cleansing themselves of invading bacteria, dead skin, and menstrual flow residue; and semen, if she's sexually active, without condoms.

Without this fresh moisture, the skin of this area will become dry and unable to protect itself, and will sustain rips, bacterial infection damage, and need medical care.

Beginning with puberty, her vagina begins washing itself by producing a

---

7 Kaufman MD, Miriam, Cory Silverberg M.Ed, and Fran Odette MSW. The Ultimate Guide to Sex and Disability. San Francisco: Cleis, 2003. (Kaufman, Silverberg, and Odette p. 52)
8 The vulva (Latin, plural vulvae or vulvas) the external genital organs of the human female, including the labia majora, mons pubis, labia minora, clitoris, vaginal entrance, glands, and vaginal orifice.

clear to whitish colored liquid flow, having a watery to sticky consistency.

This protective acidic flow, first, keeps bad bacteria in check, in order to help prevent infection.

And secondly, it protects her body from damage by sperm and semen infections; whether he has an actual infection in his fluids, or whether her body perceives his sperm as an invading infection, and thus keeps her from becoming pregnant.

Wet.

A woman becoming sexually aroused should experience increased vaginal moisture, sometimes, without ever actually knowing she is aroused, only feeling "wet."

Her vulval lips should also swell, filling with blood and becoming warmer and plumper, which many women can feel between their legs; but, not all women will notice this, and not all women have sufficient blood flood to properly inflate and prepare her for sex.

It is the same basic principle that keeps men's penises from properly inflating with enough blood flow. The surge and flow of blood to the area can often be improved in both sexes with BEFORE SEX exercises, sports activities, or prolonged, warm up foreplay.

Scent.

Also, even more so than in human men, women produce their own scent, a chemical signature wholly distinctive to her, as an individual, which also signals her current reproductive and sexual state, which scientists **(those infamous Scottish ones)** say men can, subliminally, smell her differences, between her and other women, and between one state of her and another state of her, even when not fully cognizant of it.

So, that means that you should REMEMBER that, when male hormones scream a hot need to really lay this particular woman—NOW—is probably truly saying that he senses, without thinking it out clearly, that she's fertile, NOW, and it's her time for getting pregnant[9].

So, stop and think or just glove it, regardless. Or raise it through school.

While most of our noses may have lost the ability to detect these scents at great distances, I have read of men who become sexually aroused when exposed to them. And most men and women LOVE the scent of their significant other's clothing.

In actuality, an overwashed, over douched, over hygiene sprayed vulva and vagina are UNHEALTHY; because a moist vulva with its own natural, unmasked aroma is a healthy one, for life health and for sex health.

Hold the Fish: Vulvas Can Smell or Taste Unpleasant, Because:

- When normal vaginal moisture remains in the inner folds of her vulva, or

---

[9] There has been recent (21st century) Scottish medical research which confirms this, in a basic way.

- When she's ingested excessive strong foods, or
- When she has poor air circulation around her genitals.

Clothing that's tight or made of dense materials that don't breathe are major causes of excess moisture not being able to evaporate properly.

And since bacteria adore warm, moist places, they can reproduce more rapidly in such an environment; resulting in a strong taste and odor **(that infamous "fishy smell and taste," or worse)**.

It's the **bacteria** from the air or surfaces that have touched her, like fingertips, clothing, etcetera, that're actually causing the unpleasant odor, not her vaginal moisture.

Naturally clean, naturally healthy women DO NOT SMELL LIKE BAD FISH.

If a woman does feel and is completely convinced that her genitals smell or taste bad, she should first ask her sex partner, who often enjoys and is practically hypnotized by her scent that she herself finds unpleasant.

However, if her genitals do have odor problems, it will most likely indicate the presence of a serious infection.

Some partner's, who're scent sensitive, can know even before she does that she is developing a yeast infection. She should seek a doctor's advice.

Again, the often joked about "fishy" or "yeasty" smell IS NOT NORMAL and isn't an indication of a healthy vulva or vagina, but an indication that its owner should seek medical attention.

A woman's natural, protective genital flora will change with her current menstrual state, her current level of sexual arousal, and also depend on her diet.

And some lovers can even detect these different changes by taste and/or by smell.

"Taste Yourself."

Don't be such a wuss; not you and not her.

Know how you taste, whether male or female, because I find the best way for a man or woman of any age to know what they smell and taste like, for certain, and to become familiar with their normal healthy genital scents and tastes, is to smell and taste their own fluids; especially off their fingers after finger masturbation.

A woman, especially, will notice, for her own information and confident knowledge, that her pleasant, human scent(s) and flavor(s) slightly change throughout her hormonal month, especially depending on what she eats or drinks, or what worries and illnesses she has may have influencing change, too.

And, this isn't one-sided.

Men, too, can change flavor and scents, most often with the food, drink, or smokes they put into their bodies. Excess red meats, hard drink, and smokes can sour and bitter a man's semen smell and flavor. So, white meats, fruit juices, and NO SMOKES, fellas, and you'll be more delectable, too.

Cunnilingus: Definition.

Okay. Hadn't really occurred to me, until now; but, for those who didn't know....

Cunnilingus (kun'-nih-lin'-gus) is the action of using one's mouth, normally lips and tongue, but **not teeth**, to stimulate to excitement and arouse a female's genitals for her sexual pleasure; in particular, the clitoris (klit'-ore-iss) is noted as the most sexually sensitive part of her female genitalia.

Author and sex surveyist Shere Hite noted, from her researches, that most women can achieve orgasm easily from clitoral stimulation, especially by cunnilingus[10].

This Latin term comes from an alternative Latin word for vulva (**cunnus**) and from the Latin word for tongue (**lingua**).

And just so you know, a person, who performs cunnilingus, can be called a "cunnilinguist"; which is a pretty cool title, I must say.

"Wait! What's Her Clitoris, and Where the Hell is It?"

The **clitoris** (clit) is a sexual organ present only in female mammals and, its equivalent, in male anatomy, is most in likeness and sexual reaction with the sensitive penile head. And like a penis, it can come in many sizes.

Cunt/Vulva Image

- Clitoral hood
  (covering the glans clitoris)
- Labia Minora
- Labia Majora
- Vaginal opening

[http://en.wikipedia.org/wiki/File:HumanVulva-NewText-PhiloViv.jpg] [11]

This **normally** tiny, gumdrop-like or button-like organ, at least the tiny

---

10 Hite, Shere (2004 edition). The Hite Report: A Nationwide Study of Female Sexuality. New York, NY: Seven Stories Press. pp. 11. ISBN 1-58322-569-2.
11 Edited version of en:Image:HumanVulva-NoText-PhiloVivero.jpg (which was an edit of en:Image:Image:VulvaDiagram-800.jpg), uploaded to Wikipedia Commons by Amphis, 1 Sept 2005 12:48; http://en.wikipedia.org/wiki/File:HumanVulva-NewText-PhiloViv.jpg

portion that's visible outside the body, because there's much more of it within her body, much like with the male's penis, and is positioned frontmost on the female human, hidden behind and beneath the bottommost portion of her Mound of Venus, upon which lies her triangular pubic hair area.

The exterior (outside) labia majora (major lips) of the vulva, which are covered with pubic hair, can be parted to expose the clitoris, which lies specifically just inside the front point, where the hairless left and right inner labia minora **(minor lips)** come together, normally forming a small little hill, or tucked area **(clitoral hood, much like the hood that covers a penis, before circumcision).**

This clitoral hood functions the same, it covers and protects her sensitive clitoral head.

Her clitoris/clit lies immediately before her tiny urethra opening, from which she urinates **(pees)** and which lies between the gumdrop like clit and the larger vaginal entrance.

The clitoris has a similar function as the male penis, but her clit doesn't contain interior portions of the urethra, as the penis does, nor function directly for procreation, like semen dispensing in the male.

The clitoris' ONLY job is to stimulate sexual pleasure within her.

So, with besides when taking the matter in hand, with masturbation techniques, when her clitoris is usually brought into play, cunnilingus results in MORE SUCCESSFUL FEMALE ORGASMS than with any other sexual technique.

And pleasure is good; because we all know that pleasure makes us want to have that pleasure and more pleasure again; TO HAVE SEX AGAIN.

That's good, right? Great even.

So, RESPECT HER CLIT, it makes her just as happy as a guy who loves the pleasure his cockhead gives him.

Basic Skills and Stats.

Just like in singing, and all pleasures from vocalizing, both the basic and finesse skills used in cunnilingus and individual female responses to those skills are all over the place; but, can be improved with study, relaxation, and practice.

Web cunnilingus sex author Crid Lee gives this stat:

- 88% of married women say cunnilingus is their preferred form of sexual activity.

The clitoris is the most sexually sensitive part of the female body for almost all women. **(There can be variations because of sickness, injury, or personal sensitivities.)**

- There're 8,000 nerve endings in a woman's tiny clitoris! Equal to or more—**depending on who's counting**—than on the comparatively huge head of a penis glans (4,000). Making it the most highly sensitive organ in female or male.

It surpasses other highly sensitive human body parts: the lips, tongue **(good** for you), hands, and inner thighs **(especially on a woman)**.

"Her clitoris can be too sensitive to touch...."

Okay, so with this is mind, the clitoris can, at times, be **too** sensitive to stimulate by direct touch; especially, in the early stages of your female's arousal.

So, my immediate thoughts include:
- Blowing your warm breath across her, or
- Gently touching her with something VERY soft—soft feather or silk, perhaps. Yum.
- Or, just be patient and help her warm up and "get her blood flowing," so to speak.

In case you didn't know, many women, in masturbating throughout their lives, often only apply pressure on the OUTER side of her Venus Mound, without direct touch on her clitoral area.

Or some use flat fingered friction and gentle pressure of their fingers.

So, when you start poking around with blunt; hard cock; hard nailed, rough fingertips; and hard tongues, she just may find it unpleasant.

Think the kind of unpleasantness you get when you take a bandage off a wound that's basically healed, but is still overly pink, and sensitive. You put a bandage back on it. But, she can't quite do that.

Ripping it off would be horrific!

So, basically, it all depends on how sensitive she is, how sensitive her clit is at **that** moment, and how soon you get to that area.

In fact, it's often best to begin with a gentler, less direct and straight to clit-focused stimulation of her vulval area, starting with her labial lips and the whole genital area; or the insides of her sensitive to kisses and other affection attention thighs.

Hey, my friend, she has an ENTIRE body "wonderland" for you to play with and inspire to joy; besides:
- According to Dr. Seymour Fisher in his "The Female Orgasm," of 300 **women surveyed,** 80% NEEDED masturbation or oral stimulation, also, during standard intercourse, IN ORDER TO ORGASM **(in order to come / cum)**, at all.

This is while engaging in **regular, vanilla** sex.

Yes, standard, traditional vaginal **[cock in cunt]** sex, and not during anything fancy and intimidating.

The EXACT same thing was previously confirmed DECADES before, by our famously infamous Dr. Alfred Kinsey in his thorough and still quite current "Kinsey Report" **(1948 and 1953)**, which was **the** FIRST OFFICIAL STUDY OF SEX, EVER.

Yeah. That recent. Dr. Freud made us neurotic about it, with unsupported, misinterpreted word of mouth, but didn't officially study it.

Also check out Dr. Debora Phillips' writings of her more recent "Sexual Confidence", as well.[12]

============================

"Oral sex gets around issues of..."

"Oral sex gets around issues of [uncontrolled spasms], low energy, problems with erections, positioning needs, lubrication [*which can alter genital taste*], and anything that makes penetration difficult or uncomfortable [*or painful*]."

—*The Ultimate Guide to Sex and Disability*[13]

Your Basic Oral Tools.

Your tongue's tip point, its blade side, or its flat underside or flat top can be used, as well as your nose, your chin, your lips and, with great caution, your teeth; which if shielded with your lips, as if pretending to be toothless, is usually about as hard as **most** women can stand.

But don't gum like a crazed baby, because if you've ever stupidly—**and I have**—put your finger between a babies toothless gums; I bet you NEVER did it again. It hurts; a lot. But a finger has bone inside to protect it.

Her clit, though, has more in common structurally with a soft gumdrop than a hard, bony finger.

So, again, no crazed baby stuff.

FYI: There are special teeth guards...

...to protect the genitals during oral sex; they look similar to the teeth-whitening trays worn over the teeth; or those boxing or American football players' teeth guards.

When in doubt, close your eye and poke at it with something equivalent to the pressure and hardness you wish to use on her. If you don't poke your own eye out, while it's shielded by your lid, that might be just about right for her.

Maybe.

Better too soft, she can always say, "Harder."

Hey, if you blind yourself, on her behalf, she **might feel sorry** when she finds out why, and let you have more time, uh, below.

Or she'll just think you're an idiot; because, again, it depends on your

---

12 Hayden, Naura. How to Satisfy a Woman EVERY Time ... and Have Her Beg for More! New York: Bibli O'Phile Books, Inc., 2001. And also Hayden, Naura. How to Satisfy a Man EVERY Time ... and Have Him Beg for More! New York: Kensington Books, 1999.
13 Kaufman MD, Miriam, Cory Silverberg M.Ed, and Fran Odette MSW. The Ultimate Guide to Sex and Disability. San Francisco: Cleis, 2003. (Kaufman, Silverberg, and Odette p. 151)

particular woman and your intercommunication skills and emotional link.

Cunnilingual Movements.

Cunnilingual movements can be unhurried and positively dawdling or fast and flicking; steady or erratic with changeable, unpredictable rhythms; firm and rigid or soft and light or squishy; all depending on your receiver's preferences and your tongue and lip articulation skills.

Your pleasure-giving tongue can even be inserted into her vagina, whether rigid and moving or rigid and unmoving; whichever she indicates to you is the way(s) she prefers.

And, there are tongue appliances available, for you to put over your own tongue, as an extension, or to be used on a little machine of its own; and actually flicks like a tongue, but never tires, well, at least until the batteries run out.

These are especially good for those with tongue problems, like paralysis or partial removal.

[Editor's Note, Calston:

Look for Lady Calston "The Tongue" and "Mini Tongue" by Calston Industries www.calston.com/ and other such devices from MANY companies, including leader California Exotic Novelties www.calexotics.com/.]

Also, making humming vibrations, while performing cunnilingus, is often considered exceptionally arousing and tingly; especially with certain rhythms, pitches, or songs. But you'll have to pick the one that suits you and her, I'm not telling mine.

So, my friend, what is or will be "your song," as a loving couple?

Education, Partners, and Restrictions.

Some contemporary sex educators recommend cunnilingus, as THE CHIEF INGREDIENT, when making love to a woman—**not just using it as quick foreplay**[14] **to get her ready for the "main event" of penetrative intercourse**.

Some women will find cunnilingus far too intimate, while others will love exactly that about it.

Let's literally face it, most sex, as we talk about it and see it in films and books, is all about guys. All about the dick; going in and getting hard; and spurting all over the place, and how she loves it.

Even a lot of romance stories, whether ripping bodices or not, are somewhat like this, somewhat distant and male filtered, since women, despite women's female subculture, do grow up in the same über male focused culture that men do.

There's also a whole overt and subtext thing going on about cruelty to women; including blooding them on first penetration—and **documenting** it, proving it **for all to literally see**, with **blood-stained sheets** on the following wedding morning.

---
14 Masters, W.H.; Johnson, V.E. (1966). Human Sexual Response. Toronto; New York: Bantam Books. ISBN 0 553-20429-7.

That sort of thing.

Well, this book and this subject are all about the cunt, the most female thing on the planet.

Every woman has one.

Everyone came out of one.

And when the cunt is happy, the cock gets MORE, so he'll just have to wait, for now, like waiting for fine wine; better grapes, better wine, over time.

Cunnilingus can easily be partnered with gently inserted finger(s) or an adult sex toy **[Editor's note: It's always "adult sex toy" as if you can find "children's" sex toys?]** for her vagina or anus, or both, fingers and toy; to add synchronized or unsynchronized stimulation of her famously infamous G-spot[15].

Her G-spot is a real body part and is usually a smooth flat spot or area with small flap of skin which can feel corrugated to the touch, or it's a small nub; and it's located just about an inch inside her vagina, belly button side, or, if you prefer front side between her vaginal opening and her cervix.

Also, with finger and toy action, inserting said digits, sexual plaything, or humming vibrator into her anus can work WONDERS; either of which, for many women, can PRODUCE **INTENSE, PLEASURABLE SENSATIONS**.[16]

Plus, my sexual master friend, other activities, as well, can be partnered with cunnilingus, in order to increase ALL OVER PLEASURE for both playful partners; restricted only by your mutual individual psychologies, personal preferences, and combined and individual physical anatomies.

Pregnancy.

Yes, the infamous "Nine Months Flu."

There is a potential risk of pregnancy, from mismanaged cunnilingus; especially, if semen's hardy little upstream swimmers, come in contact with the moist vaginal area indirectly.

Please, none of that we didn't "go all the way," "just did" this or that.

When fresh semen is deposited on the vulva lips, even when NOT directly placed INTO the vagina, semen can still get her pregnant.

So, be careful, unless babies are a result you both want, because if semen's precum or ejaculate, from masturbation, for instance, is carried on your or her fingertips, palms, or other part of the body **(like the tongue of a third party player, for instance)**, and comes in contact with her sensitive and moist vaginal

---

15 The Gräfenberg spot, or G-spot, is a female sexually responsive zone which, when stimulated, leads to high levels of sexual arousal and powerful orgasms. The G-spot's existence is been widely accepted by the public and most sexology books treat it as fact.

Gynecologists and other doctors continue to be skeptical of the existence of the G-spot *(which seems absurd since there's a definite spot that's touchable and different from the rest of the vagina)*.

One study of female ejaculation, 84% of the approximately 1300 professional women, who re-sponded, reported a sensitive area in the vagina, and this was connected with those reporting ejaculation.

16 Human sexuality in a world of diversity. New Jersey, USA: Pearson Education. 2005 edition. pp. 124,226. ISBN 1-205-46013-5.

SexSinger: Cunnilingus

area, there can be crying babies soon made.

Imagine the overheated situation of a threeway, and if one female **(or male)** fellates **(male oral sex/give head)** the man and then soon follows by giving the other female cunnilingus...?

Or he's doing that porn vid thing, "money shot" thingy, of jacking off onto her pubic area, vulva, or even anus. **(They're REAL close on a woman, remember? And if you didn't, go look at the real thing, a real cunt, that is, or a diagram.)**

So, it's still a great idea to be cautious, always know where your hands and tongues have recently been and are at present. Keep a moist antiseptic towel nearby, or make a trip to wash your hands a seductive part of the sex.

Virgo astrological types will **love** it.

And you're thinking "wash your hands a seductive part of sex"? Yes, "If you wash and sterilize your hands, baby, I'll _____ **(fill in the blank)** for you."

Now. What seductive little thing or activity could she possibly do in thanks to your cleanliness, **after** you've completed your cunning cunny taste task? Or **during?**

============================

"I dove. I actually dove in and licked Alice's juicy..."

"I dove. I actually dove in and licked Alice's juicy pussy, like a greedy little pig and loved it!

"She moaned louder, writhing and grinding hot and wet against my face, smothering me in plump, musky flesh, and tart juice, juice, and more juice, flowing like a river.

"I kept getting it in my nose, but I couldn't stop lapping at her and she kept moaning, as I nipped and pinched with my lips and she moaned louder. I poked my tongue hard inside her—.

"Then felt him behind me...."

—"Laila's BFF Dream" from *Neale Sourna's North Coast Academies' Diary*, Volume 1 Number 1 [NCADv1n1]; available now, ebook and/or print

----

CULTURAL, SPIRITUAL, and RELIGIOUS SIGNIFICANCE; and a BIT of LEGAL HISTORY.

No, my rightwing, hardcore religious friends, cunnilingus is **not** a **new** invention.

Artistic images of cunnilingus can be found in the long ago volcanic buried mosaics of Pompeii, Italy, which date from pre 79 AD.

And it didn't start there. People are people, no matter what time period, no matter what they SAY the conventions and laws of the area are; SOMEONE is the master expert of cunnilingus and other sexual "no-no," naughty pursuits. Which means, yes, Puritans had a lot more sex and sexual choices than most historians normally let on, which they've edited out for history classes.

If you look, the info is there.

"Worldwide Cultural Attitudes."

Cultural and regional attitudes towards oral sex, in general, yesterday and today, range from gut-wrenching disgust to hosanna singing worship, and vary greatly, depending on who is giving and who is receiving, who is of elevated social status and who is of lower, or whether same sex or one of each.

Oral sex has been utterly forbidden or at least frowned upon in many cultures and parts of the world.

Reasons often are:

- that oral sex **doesn't** lead to procreation, and that **all** sex should;
- or that it's a **humiliating** and/or **unclean** practice

This latter "unclean" opinion, at least in some cases, which some people still express today, is connected with the negative symbolism attached to different parts of the body; especially those body parts below the waist and above the knee, **but most especially if the body is female.**

Another reason in discouraging oral sex, for some, was and for many **still** is that women should **NEVER** have physical sexual pleasure; and as **much** childbirth pain, as various godly deities of yesteryear and today will allow; according to various pious "dick"-tates and fancifully error-based legalities and supposed socially-imposed "concerns."

Which usually means forcefully keeping all of **their** women and any visiting women from other cultures from having personal desires and individual sexual thoughts of their feminine own.

But that's not you or me, is it?

Freethinking women with delicious feelings we generate in them, don't frighten us.

And one last, major discouragement often expressed is when any physical "ailment" or "continuing condition" is added to the sexual intercourse mix; which can weigh against your lover's enjoyment and relaxation into her joy.

Because, when was the last time you heard anyone, or yourself, encouraging someone in a wheelchair or under constant med attention, in an institution, etcetera, to sexually enjoy themselves; as all humans, especially, adult ones have the right to do?

Hm. Yes. I thought so. Me, too.

But, such people aren't saints nor are they all emotional or completely physically sexless eunuchs. Be careful of thoughts and feelings like that, some actual eunuchs in history had children AFTER they were "fixed."

So much for faulty thinking and faulty surgical techniques.

Besides, we all know that sex and love are for EVERYONE.

Yes, everyone.

============================

"Desire and Self-Esteem."

"I spent my teen years desperately wanting something, but I didn't know what it was. I didn't think it could be sex, because when I heard [others] talking about girls, it was all about how they looked, and since I can't see girls, I figured I couldn't be attracted to them.

" 'They' NEVER talked about how [wonderful] girls smell, the way a [weighty or firm] breast feels cupped in your hand, how you feel when they whisper [delicious] things in your ears, the [incredible emotional and body] thrill of kissing....

"As you can see, I've got it figured out now, but *then*, it was just a nameless desire."

—*The Ultimate Guide to Sex and Disability*[17]

"Cultural Legalities[18]."

Around 1500 BC, the Semitic Hittite people of the Mesopotamia Region **(Iraq, Syria, Turkey)** were harshly forbidden from indulging in oral sex.

Period.

Even while married.

And such laws as the Hittite's have "remained on the books" of legal matters for many places in the world.

Not unlike many places today which still have such laws on their legal books discouraging and outlawing same sex sexual matters, unless, of course, if they're the odd sex **(male)** pleasurably watching and cavorting with the other same **(female)** sexers.

Anyway, Hittite fans, that's over 3500 years, of bad, unfulfilling, and grossly dull sex!

For centuries of women.

It's positively mind- and body-numbing.

These laws remain, still, not because anyone was abusing anyone or killing anyone, because that sort of behavior was expected, after all—**endless torture, child and wife physical and sexual abuse, lifetime slavery, and never-ending wars and beheadings were daily expectations**—however, whether heterosexual or homosexual, oral sex was off the table, as not being "sanctioned, appropriate behavior."

---

17 Kaufman MD, Miriam, Cory Silverberg M.Ed, and Fran Odette MSW. The Ultimate Guide to Sex and Disability. San Francisco: Cleis, 2003. (Kaufman, Silverberg, and Odette p. 13)
18 Birch PhD, Robert W. (1996). Oral Caress: The Loving Guide to Exciting a Woman. Columbus, Ohio: PEC Publications. p. 15. ISBN 1-57074-307-X

It was listed as "crimes **against** nature," "perversion," "moral deprivation," and "lewd **and** lascivious conduct."

Oh, yes, and "sodomy **and** gross indecency," plus "taking improper **and** unnatural liberties."

Check your **local** laws, what **you're doing in private** might still be on the books!

So, my sexy friend, feel a little pervy. Are you still with me here?

Religious Culture: Chinese Spiritual Taoism.

Cunnilingus hasn't been openly nor graciously spoken of in Western society, not until quite recently; however, it's held an honored and respected place in ancient Chinese Taoism[19]; because the ultimate aim of Taoism is to attain immortality, or at least a long life's longevity.

From ancient times, to a Taoist, the **loss** of semen, plus vaginal, and other bodily liquids is believed to encourage a reciprocal **loss** of vitality.

By retaining the male semen **(keeping it in the chute, shall we say)** or drinking the flavorful vaginal goddess-given fluids, including, sometimes, menstrual blood, too, it was believed that a man could conserve and even increase his Qi **(or Ch'i)**, or his original, spiritual living breath.

"The Great Medicine of the Three Mountain Peaks…"

"…is to be found in the body of the woman and is composed of three juices, or essences: one from the woman's mouth, another from her breasts, and the third, the most powerful, from the *Grotto of the White Tiger*, which is at the *Peak of the Purple Mushroom* (the mons veneris)."

—Octavio Paz. <u>Conjunctions and Disjunctions</u>. Trans. Helen R. Lane. 1975. (London: Wildwood House, 1969) p. 97.

According to author and teacher of Oriental Studies, Philip Rawson (in Octavio Paz, p. 97), to him, these half-poetic, half-medicinal metaphors explain the popularity of cunnilingus among the Taoist Chinese:

"The practice (of cunnilingus)…

…was an excellent method of imbibing the precious feminine fluid." (Paz, p. 97)

But the Taoist ideal is not just about the male being enriched by engorging himself with female secretions; she also benefits from her **communion** with her male.

Ideally, in fact, by intermixing the female and male generated liquids,

---

[19] Taoism (also spelled Daoism) is a variety of interrelated philosophical and religious traditions and concepts, which has influenced East Asia for over two thousand years, and is now worldwide. The Chinese language character Tao (or Dao) means "path" or "way," and has taken on more abstract meanings for more Western practitioners. Taoist ethics stress the "Three Jewels of the Tao": compassion, moderation, and humility. Taoist thought focuses on health, longevity, immortality, wu wei (nonaction), and spontaneity.

Taoists aim to balance opposites: the yin and the yang, inaction and action; and recapture the mythical, spiritual time that existed long before the full division of the sexes in the primordial time of the original **Qi**.

[**As in the Holy Bible's Old Testament, before the combined spirit man/woman was separated apart and then given individual physical bodies.**]

Culture Philosophy: Indian Tantra.

There's a similar desire, in Tantra, to transcend old age and death, and to achieve a state of perfection, total peace from all cares and pain **(nirvana)**, in the Hindu practice of Tantric yoga.

The same importance of retention and absorption of vital sex liquids in the ancient Sanskrit language **[1500 BC to today]** texts explain how the male's semen must not be discharged, if he wishes to escape the powerful laws of limited time and death.

"Songs of Solomon."

Verse 7:3 **(verse 7:2 in the Holy Bible's Old Testament, King James Version)** of the Songs of Solomon contains a fairly direct mention of cunnilingus, while most English translators, however, hysterically avoid it, by using the term "navel," instead.

Which means, the alternate, **true translation** would read as:

"Your vulva [*not navel*] is a rounded crater, never lacking mixed wine."

Which makes a hell of a lot more sense, to me, anyway.

Ah, those embarrassing Solomon Songs and his sinful sexual actions with his excessive (to God) thousand or so wives, uh, sorry (1 Kings 11:3) "seven hundred **wives (allegedly all foreign princesses)** and three hundred **concubines (just chicks he liked or were given as presents, I guess).**"

And that **these women** "led Solomon astray" from his God. Hm, he bought or received women as gifts, but THEY made **him,** a supposedly powerful and wise male king, sin?

I mean **this is the guy that put Genies in bottles!** But, he couldn't say a dick "no" or keep his excessive amount of wives and girlfriends, uh, babies' mamas under control?

Hm.

So, how many of us have this questionable tale buried in our psyches about male/female relations floating up when we're randy?

The sexual context of these sacred texts, when corrected, moves us readers following the male's point of view of his beloved from her sandals, up to her vulva, to her belly, and to her breasts; making "vulva" (Heb. **shor**), as taken from an ancient Aramaic word meaning "secret place,"[20] much more sensible; except to those of you out there who are all squeamish about **happy women having happy sex**; especially in a religious based book.

I mean, really, how many of us, who aren't fetishists, would stop at a woman's NAVEL when she's got breasts above and vulva/cunt below?

Duh, dude.

Christian and Jewish tradition, both stress spiritual, but not, for the most part, **physical** importance to the erotic intimacy between bride and groom, wife and husband that's described in the **Songs of Solomon**.

And most especially not physical erotic joy for her.

And, maybe it's just me, but the Muslims are usually neck and neck with this same tradition, stressing "beautiful virgins in paradise" **for him**, but are there ever "handsome studs in paradise" **for her?**

I think not. Or did I miss that?

=============================

"If Dara wished to allow the princess to touch her,...."

"...Tor would not deny it; though the sight of them together jolted awake the long napping, sharply cold darkness within him.

"Ahlhild was still caressing and now hungrily lapping at his Dara's womanhood, as the queen lay on her back, and the princess put her always too busy tongue to more delicate use, while inserting her tanned white fingers deep into the heated wetness of His Dara's mulberry sweet and most sacred place, in a manner that should have remained his alone to enjoy.

"The thought of snapping the white bitch's neck or shoving her from one of the high, sheer narrow paths Dara had said they had yet to pass, lingered graphically in his mind.

"He watched them, while his Bänd responded too favorably to the forward attentions of the errant—.

"The next word he used in his mind for her would have seared and shriveled Ahlhild, if he had said it to her in person, in the manner and passion it was expressed inside him.

"He mused in his axe-sharp thoughts, without amusement, that she would not hear him now, though, as her ears were now pinned between Dara's strong thighs.

"He watched and waited, and was too angered to be aroused. He watched and waited, as His Queen now rode atop the white cunt's face, as if she were riding across her great plains, until her pleasure peaked and her beautiful, sweet satisfaction overflowed from her.

"Ahlhild lapped at that, as well, leaving...."

---

20 Cf. the brief discussion in Brown, Francis; Driver, S.R., and Briggs, Charles A. Hebrew & English Lexicon of the Old Testament. Oxford: The Clarendon Press, 1902; repr. 1978; p. 1057a. A more complete discussion is found in Frants Buhl's edition of Wilhelm Gesenius' Hebräisches und Aramäisches Handwörterbuch über das Alte Testament. *[Hebrew and Aramaic Dictionary Over/of the Old Testament]* Göttingen: Springer-Verlag, 1915; repr. 1962; p. 863a.

— erotic novel work in progress "All Along the Watchtower, Book Two" by Neale Sourna

----

THE ICKY MEDICAL STUFF.

"Ew!" Yucky Stuff: STD, HPV, and Alleged Oral Cancer Risk.

ALL ORAL SEX can transmit these sexually transmitted diseases (STDs): human papillomavirus (HPV), Chlamydia, herpes, gonorrhea, hepatitis **(multiple strains)**, and other diseases, including HIV.

Any DIRECT body fluid contact with a person infected with HIV **(the virus that causes AIDS)** can give the other person a risk of that infection.

However, this is generally considered much lower than the dangerous risk associated with bare vaginal or bare anal sex, per the US Center for Disease Control (CDC).[21]

Personal STD control.

If your female receiving partner has even slight wounds, scratches, or open sore spots on or within her genitals, **for any reason,** or if you, the giving partner, has:

- slight wounds,
- scratches, or
- open sore spots,

for any reason, on or within your mouth, such as:

- bleeding gums, or
- a paper cut on the tongue or lip,

or anything such, just ONE of these, let alone, more than one combined, increases the risk of STD infectious transmission between you two.

Even just simply:

- brushing your teeth,
- flossing, or
- undergoing dental work, like
- dental cleaning, or
- eating hard, crunchy foods, like corn or potato chips,

fairly soon before or just after performing cunnilingus **(or other oral sex, for that matter)** can also increase the risk of spreading STDs and other common bacteria and viruses between you two.

---

21 http://www.cdc.gov/hiv/resources/Factsheets/pdf/oralsex.pdf *[still online at publishing]*

Or even from previous sex partners of either, or both of you!

Why?

Because all of these everyday actions make tiny, microscopic nicks and scratches in your mouth's skin lining, gums, and tongue.

And infections like bacteria and tiny viruses LOVE them. Think of it as being in a war and they find the tiniest chink in your armor, and slither and crawl through.

Oops.

"And, just so you know:"

A 2005 research study, conducted at Sweden's College of Malmö, suggested a **noticeable correlation** between **performing unprotected oral sex** on a human papillomavirus (HPV) infected person might increase risk of oral cancer.

They found that 36% of cancer patients had HPV compared, to **only 1% of the healthy control group.**

Another more recent study suggests a connection between oral sex and throat cancer[22], probably also due, again, to transmission of HPV, since it's involved in most cervical cancers.

This last study concluded that those with one (1) to five (5) oral sex partners, in their lifetime, about **doubled** their risk of throat cancer, compared with those who'd **never** engaged in oral sex, also **those with more than five (5) oral sex partners appeared to have a 250% increased risk.**[23]

Oral Sex STD Prevention.

In the matter of your health and life protection and hers, use protective dental dams[24]—**which do block genital taste and smell**—when performing or receiving oral sex, including cunnilingus, especially with a partner whose STD or other hidden illness status is completely unknown.

You can make an improvised dental dam out of a slit open condom **(search reliable med and sex sites online for instructions).**

A real dental dam is preferred by all medical professionals for sex, since dental dams are larger than condoms, and because an improvised dam can be made ineffective, when poked with scissors in their making.

Or stretched and thinned with the handling.

And, yes, urban legends and urban advice, plastic wrap can also be used, but is **less effective** because its thickness dulls sensation. Also, some plastic wraps are constructed with tiny holes which allow heat and moisture venting during

---

22 Oral sex can cause throat cancer - 09 May 2007 - New Scientist
23 D'Souza G, Kreimer AR, Viscidi R, et al (2007). "Case-control study of human papillomavirus and oropharyngeal cancer". N. Engl. J. Med. 356 (19): 1944–56. doi:10.1056/NEJMoa065497. PMID 17494927. http://content.nejm.org/cgi/pmidlookup?view=short&pmid=17494927&promo=ONFLNS19.
24 Dental dams or rubber dams are rectangular sheets of latex (or silicone) used in dentistry; and are also used during sexual activities, as a safe sex method, by being a barrier between sexual partners, in the same manner as a condom is a barrier.

SexSinger: Cunnilingus

microwaving, meaning **these same holes can permit dangerous diseases and viruses to pass between you.**

And, again, plastic wrap and such materials can be stretched and thinned with the handling, and have hidden rips. Think a condom pricked by a naughty person with a straight pin. You may not ever see the hole but someone's sperm or deadly virus will.

Warning: Dental Dam and Condom Protection.

Doing cunnilingus or fellatio or anilingus **on ANYONE you haven't specifically seen their medical files stating, "Perfect Health," without** *any* **STDs***; use a dental dam over her cunt, a condom over his dick, and a dental dam over whomever's anus between them and your mouth.*

And between your mouth and them.

STDs, like communication, move in both directions. So, whether male or female or both, carry and wear protection of your health and life, and theirs.

Always.

No, you can't trust their vowing to whatever gods and their live mother's grave that they're clean and uninfected.

Yes, you lose taste and smell and skin to skin barebackness, but some sexually transmitted diseases NEVER go away; **not until you die***. Soon.*

Popular Culture and Slang.

There are numerous slang terms for cunnilingus, including "drinking from the furry cup," and "muff-diving."

In lesbian culture, several common slang terms have been "giving lip," "lip service," or "tipping the velvet" **(an expression novelist Sarah Waters is said to have "plucked from the relative obscurity of Victorian porn").**

[Victorian Porn = lots of beating with tree switches and/or incest of varying degrees, school sex, and sex with virgin women from all around the world fantasies. See the Victorian underground newsletter, "The Pearl"][25]

Such elderly erotic literature refers to cunnilingus as "gamahuching" **[gah' mah hoosh' ing]** or "gamahuche," with some spelling variations.[26]

"Frank and Louisa are too busy to notice what we...."

"Frank and Louisa are too busy to notice what we do," I whispered in her ear, as I inclined the willing girl *[his cousin, first cousin, I think, so she's close as a sister but legally and morally "okay"]* backwards on the soft pillow of sand, and reversing my position, we laid at full length, side by side, both of us as eager as possible for the game; my head was buried between her loving thighs, with which she pressed me

---

25 1880, Anonymous, The Pearl: A magnum opus of Victorian erotica (1996)
26 1880, Anonymous, The Pearl: A magnum opus of Victorian erotica (1996)

most amorously, as my tongue was inserted in her loving slit; this was fine gamahuche.

— "The Pearl" [*an under ground erotic newsletter, 1880*] **edited by Carroll and Graf Staff, James Holmes, Carroll & Graf, 1996**

And, if you didn't already know, cunnilingus is also called "eating out" or "poon-job"; a slang term and cunnilingus variant of the fellatio/male-centered slang term "blowjob."

"Poon" is short for poontang[27] or punani, among **many, many, many** other terms, which would go on for pages and pages.

You can see reference materials in footnotes/Endnotes, if you're interested; and of course you are.[28]

The phrase "cunning linguist" is also often used as an oral pun; which is "clean enough" for mainstream American television.

And, supposedly, at one time, a Hell's Angel motorcycle club member, "whose colors includes red wings, indicates that he or she has performed cunnilingus on a woman, while she was on her period or black wings for performing cunnilingus on a black woman.[29]

What? No wing color, striped, checkered, or plaid, for a black woman on her period?

Or perhaps black wings, lined with red?

Or what color for lapping a Native American, or half Native American half African American, on her period?

And yes, friends, I can go on for days with this train, or is it tranny **[transsexual]**, of thought?

MASTERING SexSinging BASIC ARTISTIC SKILLS.

Always remember that, contrary to what some doofuses think, believe, and say, "**Every** woman," is NOT, "the same," but **different**, so **vary** your style, speed, and force when performing oral upon the particular individual her you are with.

Think of it as singing or performing a song, you wouldn't do the **same** old **one** song over and over and over and over again, would you?

But, if **you** would, what song could that possibly be, that was THE **only** song; with all the **same** tune, **same** ups and downs, and **same** speeds, that you'd want for the rest of your long life?

Or that she'd want? Over and over and over and...?

---

27 Poontang [From French putain "whore"]—(1) *(US, colloquial noun, vulgar)* Female genitalia; the vulva or vagina. Also: poon, tang, pussy, punani, cooch, coochie, cunt, gash, slit, snatch, twat, pink taco. (2) *(US, slang verb, vulgar, uncountable)* Sexual intercourse with a woman. As in, "I gotta get me some poontang tonight." Also: poon, tang, pussy, punani, ass, tail

28 Green, Jonathon, and Kipper Williams (cartoons). The Big Book of Filth: 6500 Sex Slang Words and Phrases. 4th Edition. London: Cassell, 2003. Print. And Dalzell, Tom, and Istvan Banyai (illustrator). The Slang of Sin. 1st Ed. Springfield, Massachusetts USA: Merriam-Webster Inc, 1998. Print.

29 Thompson, Hunter S. (1995). Hell's Angels. New York: Ballantine Books. pp. 64. ISBN 0-345-41008-4.

SexSinger: Cunnilingus 27

Learning to Play—Your Way.

Also remember, it's the way **you** individually do what **you** and only **you** can do, **in your own particular way**.

Her pussy is your instrument.

New Orleans born musicians the late Louis Armstrong and the very alive Wynton Marsalis are trumpeters, and yet they both play fabulously well, but not EXACTLY the same.

You can tell by your ears, and how each makes you feel, and she can tell you from another, by your tonguing.

Be sexy about it.

Okay, let's clarify that a little better. Don't be what and who you misbelieve is tough movie sexy or adventure sexy or porn film sexy.

No. Really. Don't.

Be you. Because she chose to be **with you**, and well, also know that...

...when she's open like that, she really is a delicate flower, opening and exposing her most tender, vulnerable petals **to you**.

So, I guess that really does make you her bee. And bees get **all** the honey; well, pollen in actuality. You get my point.

Just don't be all busy and fast and all over the place like real bees.

Okay, let's leave bee land.

A Bit More on Women's Social History.

Little girls, worldwide today and historically everywhere, are or have been expected to remain close to home and literally inside the home, away from all men not direct relatives, and demanded, to be always neat and clean from the very moment they're born.

Little boys, however, are expected to go outside and are easily forgiven when they go leave home and get dirty and explore, but girls still often must ruthlessly maintain the cleanliness of their personal clothes and body; even the ones who look sloppy with a fully fashioned, disheveled look.

Girls are still taught to ALWAYS look as attractive—**no matter how disheveled, again, think sexy bed head hair, for instance**—and smell as sweet and clean and floral as possible.

And for god's sake, girly, DON'T SWEAT or dare to have hairy legs or a stray wisp found in your armpits! As a recent world famous woman singer was abused about recently because of a few stray strands of pit hair.

Female with hairy-ish pits? You'll make every vicious, giggling online and broadcast gossip blog edition.

With scary zoom, in HiDef.

Boys and men, too, rarely are required to be so clean, and the ones who do by natural inclination are suspect as being less manly than his dirty, sweaty, smelly brothers.

And NBA Cavalier LeBron James' hairy male pits are prominently placed on a building sized poster over the central main entrance into Cleveland town.

Without comment, except from me, of course.

Many, many women have the freakish, personal clean body mentality and the idea that a woman's natural scents and functions of sweating, even when doing strenuous activities on a hot day, and such **are foul and wrong and positively sinful,** as if further evidence of Lucifer's wicked hold on the wicked Daughters' of Eve.

"Dirty Girl"—character Baby Stewie, TV's "Family Guy."

Give more awareness and heartfelt, thoughtful consideration to the negative shame-inducing energies attached to "feminine hygiene," and its products; especially in ads and marketing.

This excessive personal feminine hygiene attention leads people to subliminally and downright blatantly believe that natural ANY scent or wetness coming from the female body, is horrendous, improper and needs to be corrected, hidden, and not really talked about.

But, perhaps, laughed about. And, it's funny, until it's your sister or the one you want to love.

Lets face it, where are all the relentlessly played ads for masculine "deodorant sprays" or "masculine washes" for removing that smell and unsavory, curdled cream from unsanitary cheesy dicks **(y'know, there's always that one guy in class, whether in gym or out).**

Or that "embarrassing" male drippage, that "problem" sweaty balls, and "secret" male genital itchiness called "jock itch," which US TV advertised a product for a brief while, back in the 70s, then nearly immediately pulled it off air.

But, the female equivalents have persisted and multiplied to the embarrassing point of having to sit through three of four or five of them back to back to back, while we sit watching TV with a member of the opposite sex we're interested in.

It's a lie, you know, to make sales bucks, but it burns into a person's mind; making women believe and feel they're dirty "down there" and some men paranoid to believe and feel that women really are dirty overall, as well.

"Evil and dirty."

With nearly everyone saying that natural female body scent is "odor," it's no huge surprise that many clean women truly believe they have "dirty, smelly genitals" that no one would ever truly want to put their face into.

When, in fact, these wonderful women have perfect and normal and extremely healthy sex organs; plenty faces want to get into.

But, you may have to help her with that, so you can help her have fun.

=============================

"He stared between my legs, as he slid…"

"He stared between my legs, as he slid one of my legs high over his broad shoulder.

"He bent down and kissed me, on my clit! *many* times, and licked, and licked, and sucked on me, until I thought I'd die, over and over again, and something, I don't know what to call it, grew in me. Can you really, truly die from physical pleasure, like this?! "

— "Laila's First Cunnilingus" from *Neale Sourna's North Coast Academies' Diary*, Volume 1 Number 1 [NCADv1n1]; available now, ebook and/or print

----

HELPING HER RELAX and PREPARE.

Don't make it a long, harsh campaign, but here are a few things to help you help her to relax and prepare for your ecstatic, pleasurable cunnilingus fun for two.

"Prolonged Foreplay/Diddling. Or Fun, Creative Stuff!"

Start with the simple, sensual, and kind stuff.

Brush her hair.

Give her a gentle head and neck massage.

Touch and caress all her erogenous zones, such as: skin, lips, spine, neck, shoulders, etc.

But do stay away from the more racy bits, like buttocks, thighs, and breasts, until she's warmed up to you and how you're making her feel with the less sexualized bits of her.

Better yet, make your seduction an all day affair, with sexy phone calls, text messages, snail mail cards or letters, if you REALLY planned ahead, email, flowers, horseback riding or other things she, as an individual, loves and is excited about can prepare her all day to be with you.

Without protest.

You may even have to go to the opera. Or cuddle up and watch female talk television, instead a male sports / news / add useless banter type here television.

But, she's worth it, to you.

But also, do be careful. Job place IT departments do monitor ALL emails and such on their company equipment; so, watch what you say in your love messages sent through company owned lines.

"Kiss Her. Long. And Deep."

Lips and tongues are sensual and have TONS of nerve endings; so, your tongue in her mouth is a forewarning of possible other places you can put your long, fat tongue.

Or your other **long** body parts.

Take your time, though, just sticking your tongue immediately into her maw will FEEL LIKE A RAPING INTRUSION, if she's not warmed up to you yet.

So, take the time to kiss her long and unhurried and deep, and you can often reap the reward of getting quite far with just kissing alone.

But, don't be too sloppy, or uptight and hurried. She'll sense it, she'll feel put upon with her entire body and will shut you down.

"Be Kind, Unwind."

Be gentle and loving with your flesh upon hers, and in hers.

Be kind to her body and yours.

Be patient with the quality time needed to make true beauty with your bodies together.

Plus, have fun, make her laugh—a belly laugh.

And be open to your nervousness and her fears, open to her discomforts and your own urgencies, and to her embarrassment and your own.

For your **own** feelings.

And for her tender or overpowering feelings, because you will most likely touch emotions and feelings in her that, perhaps, NO ONE has **ever** touched, or touched **quite right** or quite just **the wonderful way you do.**

Be kind; let her unwind, before you wind her up to....

Just so you know, there are women, who truly DON'T believe that ANY man could want to or enjoy doing cunnilingus, they ACTUALLY believe that ONLY horrid, nasty, selfish, sluts—**insert dated stereotypical term here for "bad, evil women"**—demand such a filthy thing of their men.

"Rapacious whores."

"Harlots."

"Slatternly sluts."

Well, you get the dated picture.

Or, they truly believe men only do cunny duties to lamely reciprocate for blowjobs. Well, some women do, but not most. But, be careful if your woman of choice is one of these.

She's a "good girl" to the max, and may prove a bit of a problem, for you to relax and encourage her enjoyment.

Just be forewarned, and think of author Stephen King's favorite horror character mom in **Carrie.**

Okay, here's hoping and praying that **your** girl's not that far out there.

Retooling Your Senses. With Her Stuff. (nonfetish)

These particular women are missing the point that is so very obvious to you...

...that your enjoyment of her, is truly that.

You enjoy HER; all of her, her body, her touch, her tastes, her scents, **everything**. And of course her mind and heart and soul, and all that mushy stuff, too.

But, maybe, you need a bit of practice in softening your approach to her, and sharpening your own sensitivities and sensuality. Because these two things are more than crying one boo-hoo tear when she's around or thinking she's cute and hot, FOR YOU, in an uncomfortable, crack drying g-string.

This is about her.

Say it, "About her."

Think it, "About her."

It's your mantra, "About her. Om."

Your prayer, "About her. Amen."

Try this, though, when she's not around; so, you won't feel on the spot, and because, depending on your girl, she may think it looks a little odd. And, if she has you arrested, you can show them these paragraphs.

Unless, of course, you really **do** deserve to be arrested. Hm?

Anyway, do this:

Game: Your Sensitivity to Sensuality.

If you have access to her closet and dresser, don't get creepy, but think of her and use your fingers, on several objects, try just three or four; something like a soft cotton camisole, a prickly lace bra, a slick silk slip, a woolen or raw silk dress.

Now, lay them out, and close your eyes, and keep them closed, for now, as you pick them up and examine each, separately, using your other senses, for the next five minutes or more.

- What does each feel like and how are they different?
- Besides your fingers, touch each to the flesh at the crook of your elbow, and the flesh behind your ear along your neck, or any other place on your body that might be more sensitive to softness and prickliness.

I'm not suggesting you touch your own private sexual parts with her stuff—**arrested, remember?**—but get a real **feel** for how **different** and **pleasurable** her stuff is to yours.

Much like her body stuff is different from yours.

And **fully focus** on them, and you'll be **fully focusing on her** stuff, her body; after practice.

Okay, now:

- What do her garments smell like, like her or cleaning products? Both?
- How are they different in scent?
- Do you smell perfume AND her?
- Do you smell her AND that spilled coffee scent still there?

Now, doing it alone was a dry run for you to get rid of your inner weirdness or freak outs. Or giggles, at "doing something SOO stupid." It's not, sensuality is never stupid; but it can be ignorant or blind and miss the beauty found in all its many complicated and different bits, parts, textures, and scents.

Or tastes.

No. Don't **taste** her clothes. Not unless.... I think that's a different book topic.

Game: "Sensitive Sensuality, for Two." **With Her Stuff. (still nonfetish)**

Ask her to play our game with you, to pick out items she loves for you, then to bring you in, with your eyes closed, or blindfolded—**you're sneaky and might peek a look through your lashes.**

She'll hand you items to experience and, as you do, remember to SAY what you feel. Aloud, like this, for her sake:

"Ah. This is that slinky dress; you always drive me crazy with. You look so great, but other men look at you so much.

But don't lie, but make it good.

Or fun.

Or both.

Then....

Open your eyes and tell her the important stuff, and let your emotions show in your eyes and face and voice.

"Hm, it still smells like you, wonderful, and like that great cologne I got you."

Or, less frilly.

"Hm, still smells like you, and that cologne I got you."

The point here is to short circuit any mental editing you or she might be doing, because as you really smell her things and really take in and enjoy her scent, she'll most likely hear it in the subtle tones of your voice.

And, for her to understand through a less flesh on flesh manner that YOU LOVE and ADORE HER SCENT(S). No lie.

Plus, when you finally do look at her, in this game, if you truly feel something wonderful for he, she'll **see** that and **feel** it to, from your eyes' expression.

Y'know the "windows of your soul." Your eyes and voice matched in adoration for her.

It's a win-win solution, my friend.

But, if you hate that perfume, or are less than wowed with it, tell her so. Because she will have seen your reaction on your face when you did sniff it—your eyes were closed, hers weren't. They were fixed on you, the entire time, in anticipation.

So, don't lie.

Eyes and voice should match; love-love is win-win.

Mixed matched attitude and voice, voice and eyes, or whatever will seem lukewarm and she'll become lukewarm, too.

So, don't lie.

All right, what you should get from all this is that you really need to let her SEE and HEAR how much YOU LOVE her scent and tasting her and giving her pleasure.

And control.

Control, whether having it or giving it, is ALWAYS sexy. Period.

If you start early with letting her know how wonderful she smells, how erotic her scent(s) are to you, and that the very sight and touch and delicious scent of her, even with her clothes on, and in a nonsexual situation, brings you to joy, she'll be more likely to believe you later, when she's naked, and literally open to you.

So, let her **really** know—**but not to the point of making her sick of it with your fawning and forcing her to think you're not sincere and are only lying**.

Let her know that she is truly **the** best flavor of all scents and soon tastes you enjoy.

It's scientifically proven even, because the senses of smell and taste are always married together. Lose one and the other loses its power, too. Food with no scent is yucky. And some of the best scents in the world make our mouths water.

Hm. Hot apple pie.

And if she still balks, saying it's "not clean," tell her that together you both will fix that, and then pour a lovely, warm bath for her, with or without bubbles, with music and whatever she loves, like scented candles and flowers.

And you.

Naked.

And wet.

What's not to love **here?**

Game Interruptus: Weekend Scents.

Take a weekend together, alone. No kids, no pets, no friends and family, and no deodorant or antiperspirant. Wash or shower before you leave, but leave your pits and crotches alone, no perfumes, no special crotch scent killers, either. You can take your toothbrush, but can cut or modify the use for it and toothpaste as well. It's just one weekend, a longer one is better.

The game here is that you'll have to deal with your own scents and with your lover smelling you. We wear so much scent to mask or obliterate our own, from scalp and hair cleaners, scalp moisturizers, hair gels, sprays, moisturizers, toothpaste AND mouthwash, face moisturizers and shaving gel and/or aftershave.

And that's just from the hairline to chinline, and I probably missed a few that you use, every day.

Each with its on little scent; layered and layered over your own.

Women especially can be leery of doing this kind of weekend—no one ever encourages women to be natural around their men, they should always "be picture perfect and flawless." Many are terrified of being sweaty and showing it.

Get over it.

LET GO, and sweat and smell for the weekend, together.

Okay, you can wipe your pits if you get too reeky or have to go to the store for groceries, but REALLY let yourself and your partner get a wiff of the real you.

Smell is a major part of compatibility, but if you've been masking it ALL the time...?

Do you love and like each other enough to have each other unmasked, pure, and undilitued?

Now, back to wet, clean loving.

Two Hours.

Really, just draw her a hot bath and then tell her, gently, that you will be the gentle boss of her, and that she has no cares or worries, as you "take charge" of her "relaxation and pleasure for the next two hours."

"Two hours?" she'll ask, much as you're asking now.

"Yes, at least," I say, and you will when she asks. Smile **(as I'm doing, now)** and help her get naked and wet, in the hot bath, that is.

Why, because this, on the practical level, takes care of several things, as promised:

- Her cleanliness issues

If her mom or nun at her old school had stressed all her formative years that women's "business" is all foul and dirty, then finding out now that a bath is **never** going to fix that, can tell you a lot about her.

- The hot bath will invigorate her lovely flesh.

Sex, good sex cannot happen without blood-flushed and filled genitals; this goes for a man's hard on and also for a woman's functional enjoyment, as well. The heat and any touching beneath the water line will send blood to her genitals. And this, my friend, is good.

- She'll relax.

Ask her or surprise her, by slipping into the bath once she's relaxed.

Make her laugh.

Ask her if she's seen those sexy film bath scenes with Angelina Jolie and Antonio Banderas, in "Original Sin" **(2001, go Unrated folks)** or....

Actually make an erotic video clip disc of your or her favorite naughty love and erotica scenes, and watch together. Hey, you're in hot water, make it really useful.

So called "porn" can work, but only if you're ABSOLUTELY certain she likes the porn you've picked.

And no explosions and fight scenes and car crashes, unless her favorite scenes are from David Cronenberg's erotic fetish/psychological "Crash" **(1996/7)** or such films and they **REALLY** TURN HER ON.

Otherwise you'll get excited but probably NOT in an erotic and relaxing way, and, yes, we will be having relaxing, fun sex.

Which is our goal today or night. Or both.

And always go NC-17 or XXX if you can, unless, of course, the R-rated version is the one that gets her totally hot and wet. Sometimes the R one **is** the Right one.

Be into it, be passionate, and above all, be receptive to her body language and what she asks you to do and responds to.

And why the "two hours"?

It'll give you a reasonable time to relax and not plan or hurry to do anything else. You may take longer, you may take a little less, but knowing that it'll be at least two quality hours together, will be like a hypnotic command, which it technically is, and make it easier for:

- Her to automatically **relax**, and for
- You to **not hurry** to get her where you want her to go.

Um, let's rephrase that, you're not going anywhere, but you do want to **give** her what you want to give her; some lovely tongue service.

More Cleanliness Issues.

While you're lighting candles in your bathroom and washing her hair for her, or whatever is relaxing and intimate between you in the bath area, remember, not the same old thing in the same old way because variety is your goal, too, well **one** of your goals.

No same old songs. We have some that are our favorites, but not just "Stairway to Heaven" each and EVERY time.

Your MAIN objective, during clean time, is to let her truly know how very much you're interested in pleasing HER, and her alone; so don't do the EXACT same thing for your lead up to cunnilingus every time, as if you might do it for everyone, or that you think it's a magic key that, when always repeated, **always open her legs.**

Women hate that!

So, if mindless, soulless repetition without heart is your thing and exact programs of gestures and actions that're **always in the same form** are your forte, know that she'll know, that **every** time you bathe with her or do her toenails, you expect to eat oyster.

Some may like it, most women won't.

But, then, again, if you always clean her bathroom and run the vacuum as a sign of cleanliness that truly appeals to her, well, then negotiate a fine fee for your services, friend.

Misc. on Pubic Hair: "To Be or Not to Be"—from William Shakespeare's "Hamlet"

Hair is a personal thing. It's a cultural thing. It's a generational thing. Hair is not dirty, just because it's present; it is dirty, however, when it's NEVER washed.

And EVERY hair on a woman's body seems to be of someone else's nosy, belittling concern.

Many couples find the activity of trimming or shaving her pubic area **(or his, for that matter)** is a good bit of foreplay, which encourages cunnilingus.

Some women find cunnilingus more enjoyable and personal hygiene easier when clean shaven. But, do know that sex, even a soft lick of a tongue, may have to wait a few hours or a day, after the pain of shaving or waxing subsides. Or not, depends on the lady.

Some couples prefer a full growth of pubic hair.

Some women prefer to cleanly shaved, because it seems the "it" thing, the fashionable thing, the thing they believe all lovers of cunt want today. But, will discover that some lovers find a clean-shaven vulva is too childlike to hold their interest.

In fact, it may make a woman's lover feel like an utter pedophile, which is not sexy, boys and girls. So, do keep this in mind; before it stops your fun, until the grass grows back in.

If the hair issue is an issue, whether having it or not having it, you'll need to discuss that out BEFORE you get to relaxing and burning candles and playing your soft music.

You Massage Her, Sensually.

Some women **adore** gentle massages and it'll make them feel mentally and physically relaxed and ready for more intimate touching.

But, and there always is a but, it seems, some women **don't** like to be massaged, or at least some are highly sensitive to being sexually manipulated for sex, so go with the flow of the woman you're with, and be flexible.

She may just hate others doing it to her, but adore your touch.

And just not to make you think that ALL women will have hang-ups or will be timid, there will be **many** who know **exactly** what they want, and what they need.

And it won't matter to them if there's clean or dirty, or hair or baldness.

And they'll tell you or direct you in their straightforward way, even **command** you where to go and what to do.

Good luck with that, and with it all, with all the different ladies of the cunny smorgasbord.

============================

"Feed me your cunt."

My pleasure, and yours.

In seconds, his lips pinched, and his tongue circled, licked, and poked my oyster, as I deliciously slid around on his —.

Oh, shit! Told you, no two men are —.

I became gluttonous, entirely selfish, and ground myself hard into him, tugging his head by his thick, black hair, until vising his handsome face between my thighs.

Holding your breath is a good thing, men. You want us to do it, while you're shoving your dick down our throats and we want it, too, while we're riding the Hell out of your sweet, prickly faces.

I nearly drowned him in cunt juice, finally opening my legs, so he could breathe and I could continue sliding around on his drenched mouth, that continued lapping and nipping at me, as his hot hands soared all over my exposed, flushed, and sensitive flesh.

—*Artemis with new lover Ren, her lover's brother*, from erotic novel work in progress "Aegis" by Neale Sourna

----

IN A HURRY? DON'T BE, OKAY, START HERE THEN.

Remember, don't be or, at least, appear greedy and rushed, and a pussy snob. She has an **entire** body that needs love and attention, and her lovely body is highly sensitive and all there, for you to explore and get to know how to please.

Once, you've taken an extended and fully involved tour of **all** of her....

Start in her lap, by breathing over the flesh of her Mound of Venus **(her pubic area, if you're still lost)**. And breathe your breath over her thighs, as well.

Kiss her normally **very sensitive** inner thighs, soft and gently at first

You can sniff and kiss and lick her thighs and suck **(think a few gentle "love bites"**[30]**)** in different places.

Run your tongue upward, along each lovely thigh, towards her vulva, but don't touch it, not yet. Kiss her Mound of Venus **(mons pubis, her pubic area)** and lick—which can be easier when shaved or waxed; but not necessarily more fun, especially if you're scent sensitive.

Pubes, like soft armpit hair, hold her wonderful scent close to its source; leading you in. Into her.

Hm, that sounds good.

Now, prepare.

Make certain your mouth and tongue wet and slippery.

Yes, Make Your Mouth and Tongue Wet and Slippery.

When your teasing makes her **moan** or **gasp** and **squirm** a little, or she asks you to directly lick her vulva; it's time to place your head between her thighs, and put your lips and tongue directly over her clitoris; if she hasn't already eagerly shoved your head down there.

Softly lick the clitoris, keeping your mouth wet, and do so slowly, without much force. You're just teasing, just barely. The wetness keeps the feeling sensual and slick; dry, though, is more like when a cigarette gets stuck to a lip, not pleasant.

Kiss her, right there, on her clit.

Kiss her cunt passionately, in the intense and loving way you kiss her beautiful mouth.

Then, begin caressing and stroking her there with your lips and tongue.

Don't forget her sensitive inner thighs and to kiss and lick her vulva labia **(vulva lips)**, so that you're not just kissing and licking one area to numbness. She'll quickly get bored with that.

Think about it, but **feel** it through, too.

She can't ever beg you to come back and kiss and lick and gently suck her clit, if you **never** wander off to other sensitive parts.

It's the contrast and variety, like of warm and cold kisses, or the highs and lows of music, when a great musician changes musical keys, or switches to another line of song lyric of the song sung, then goes back **to home**, to the catchy chorus, **to her clit**, which will **feel soo good**.

To her.

And to you, too.

---

[30] A love bite or hickey/hickie is a temporary mark or bruise on one's skin *(medically, a minor hematoma)* from kissing or sucking or biting forcefully enough to burst blood vessels beneath the skin. They last approx. 4–12 days. Supposedly, you can fix one by placing a frozen spoon or ice held to the site; probably as soon as possible. Or, by rubbing it with vitamin K and/or taking more Vitamin C.

[Editor's Note: Maybe you can turn this into a Hickey/Vitamin Game between you.]

Giving and sharing pleasure is always a great feeling.

Lick and kiss her vagina opening, as well, and slip your tongue into her. If she likes that, slip your tongue repeatedly in and out of her, using your tongue like a gentle cock.

Do it with purpose, but don't hurt her.

Don't Bash and Butt Your Hard Face into Her!

If she allows you to, go on the move to kiss and lick her ass cheeks. You both can try moving around each other, like you'd do when dancing, and can rub your bodies skin to skin, flesh to flesh; standing together, lying down side by side together, or on all fours, in various combinations.

Lick her wonderful assets from behind, for instance, with her on all fours, or gently bent over something that exposes her vulva to you.

Do make certain she's not bent over something with a hard edge cutting into her diaphragm, it'll hurt—**unless, of course, she likes that for the moment**—and it'll cut her breathing, making it shallow.

Shallow breathing is bad for sports, even sex sports; because no breath equals no endurance and no fun. She needs deep breaths in her lungs and blood flowing hotly to her clit, vulva, and vagina to have all the fun you're helping her have.

I suggest kissing and licking her ass, but not so much licking and kissing between her ass cheeks to her anus; especially, since her clit, vulva, and vagina are your main course here.

And, because it's far *too easy to transfer harmful bacteria with your lips and tongue, from her anus to her vagina or urethra,* **which both lead deep within her, to vulnerable uterus and fallopian tubes or bladder and kidneys**.

And, let's face it, giving her a *two week (if she goes to her MD), uncomfortable infection in her "unmentionables,"* or a lifetime of a life-threatening STD, especially if during her first time(s) at cunnilingus, probably won't win you any re-invitations to dine.

Stick to her Mound of Venus **(her outer, surface pubic area, her fun and furry and easily visible, full frontal triangle area)** and her vulval area **(clit to vagina/perineum)**.

You can always be a bit stealthy and just "kiss her ass" a short while, but not freaking her out in her mind—**if she sounds or actually stiffens**—get away from there.

She may be AFRAID that you're zooming in to ass sex, and not be ready for that, which is why WE KISS HER ASS and RETURN back to the main show, up front.

But, hang in their, my butt fans, you can come back to her backside when you're completely done, and **she's fully satiated** and give her ass and anus kisses and licks.

This will tease and test to see if she might want more, but do so gently, letting her know you love ALL of HER body and want to pleasure ALL of HER, in **every** way.

And that you aren't just an ass freak, out for one thing, behind her where she can't see your face and eyes; mud pie lover.

Many women **love, positively adore—BUT NOT ALL**—being licked from vagina to clit, in one long, loving, and luscious lick.

And don't scrimp on the kisses. Never scrimp on the basic, "I Love You, Baby, kiss"; whether soft or full soul-stirring.

But, remember, whether its kissing her ass, or licking her like a dog in love with her ice cream, **if she reacts negatively**, by squirming AWAY from you, pushing you away, or making sounds or words that sound less than positive, rah-rah!, and the like—STOP.

Yes, if she says, "Stop." Stop.

And even if she's a say the opposite of what she means girl, she'll correct you, and get you back to the cream lick.

Vanilla. Chocolate. Or Strawberry. **Neopolitan.**

Or more precisely, while loving her, and she expresses definitely dislike or disquiet, just move onto something else, and continue another bit of tonguing on another spot.

Preferably, GO BACK to one she liked **before** trying to move on. However….

When She Reacts Well to Your Action. Repeat It.

When **she reacts positively**, to a certain thing you do, **repeat it**.

And when she begins to enjoy what you're doing, start an easy rhythm, but not completely predictable and repetitive one, as you lick her. And kiss her. And gently suck her. And LOVE her.

NEVER silently guess in your mind what she **might** like the best, just ASK HER! Be her like her optometrist.

"Do you like that?"

"Is this better?"

"How's that feel?"

"Which you like better; THIS or THIS?"

Or, if she is really quiet or shy and doesn't answer, the BEST thing you're doing is whichever makes her the **loudest**, despite herself, **as she sighs, moans, whines, or whimpers** with apparent pleasure, that you're causing.

This is good, my friend. Excellent, in fact.

Now repeat it.

Repeat it.

Repeat it.

You're making contact with her, with rhythm and motion. Just like music.

Ups.

Downs.

Swirls.

Repeat.

You can put your neck and head to work, but **gently**, by using the movement of your whole head. Wag it back and forth, up and down.

Get into it, enjoy it, but don't get into it too hard and bashing.

Remember, she can feel not just your tongue and lips against her, but the warmth from your head, your hair moving against her, your cheek stubble and whiskers against her inner thighs.

Or your mustache rubbing against her mustache, or her sensitive, bare sexual skin.

Or your lively breath.

A multitude of sensation right in her lap, ah, crotch; but against her unprotected flesh.

So, use your head in sweeping motions, up and down or side to side, and constantly repeating the motion.

Caress her; with tongue, lips, and don't forget your hands and the rest of her lovely body.

Swirl your tongue around her.

Pat at....

Lap at ... her clit and the immediate area, again and again.

And, if your ears aren't blocked by her thighs, you'll hear her breathing rhythm changing, deepening, sighing, or the other sounds she makes when aroused; that signal what you're doing is really getting her and her body into it.

So, again and again, until your lady begins to twitch, jerk, or shudder. Or moan, sigh, or whatever she does.

When She's More Warmed Up.

When your lovely lady is warmed up and enjoying what you're doing more, you can be firmer with her.

No. Not disciplining her. Not unless that's what you two love to do.

What I mean is that some women love to be tongued and kissed hard, with lots of force and pressure—like on a romance novel cover, some love it fast or even super duper fast—**like NASCAR girls, but most seem to like it soft and delicate**—y'know, flower petal soft and soft kisses for soft cheeked babies.

And do that, be delicate.

Kiss her and tongue her, as if she's delicate between her thighs, in her most delicate area, because most women are.

And because thinking this way and feeling she is delicate and needs to be cherished, like the priceless person she is, will make your kisses and licks SAY exactly that.

Without one word.

Remember, her sexual organs are a hidden cove, a very tender area that normally isn't handled harshly, slapped, punched, bitten, or used roughly. It usually isn't rubbed by wool and leather and pebbles on the ground, like the rest of her body moving through life in clothes or barefoot.

So, don't be "a brainless, heartless bull in a china shop" of delicates and bang your face and teeth too hard against her tender flesh, once you're in your rhythmic motion.

Or she had my full approval to coax your doctor to do the same, the next time you need to "bend over and cough."

Vary your rhythm, if she likes that.

Or, keep your rhythm "As Is," if she says anything, like, "Stay, don't stop, just like that. Yeah."

Right?

You're **teasing** and **urging** her to orgasm, **not forcing her** and **not beating** her poor little clit up. It's a softish, smooshie-ish, living gumdrop; smooshier, so remember, **it's still attached to her, is alive,** and is full of MORE nerve endings, than any other part of her body.

And remember, it's **her** NOT her tasty gumdrop that is your highest and MOST IMPORTANT intention and focus. You're here for **her reaction, her emotional and physical reaction,** not just diddling with her **body parts.**

If you are, that's not why I'm helping you and you're on your own, when she kicks you in the head. And she can, and I'd suggest she does, at this angle, hard.

And, furthermore, just to add to your confusion on sticking with your rhythm and being gentle, some women, when they're cumming[31], like variations in your rhythms to keep them cumming; but, in general, though, when she begins to throb or shiver or quake or whatever your milady does—DON'T STOP.

On the other, less gentle hand, there are some women who will want you to make your activity harder **(or softer)**, as she orgasms **(cums/comes)**.

Or, for you to suck or nibble on her a little.

So play gently with her gentle parts and maybe she'll not be twisty with your parts that don't twist well. Not unless she asks you to be less gentle, or you ask and she agrees.

And if you are going for coercion or hard play playtime, do arrange a "safe word" between you to signal "go" and another for "stop," and maybe one for "surprise me," for any of that sort of mutually agreed on fun.

And one last also, a few women will want you to just leave them alone, as

---

31 Cumming—You may have been wondering why I normally use the spelling of cum, cumming, etcetera instead of standard English like come, coming, etcetera; my reason, is that too many times the prudish standard gets confusing. If "will you be coming soon, so we can do some hot cumming together, when we get there," I don't want any doubt about it. It's a special word for a special function.

they cum.

But, **most** will **love** for you to JUST KEEP DOING WHAT YOU'RE DOING until they're completely done.

"Get Up and Do It, Again. Amen."—lyrics, Jackson Browne's "The Pretender"

Once she's done; collapsed or exhausted or just "feeling floaty delicious" and "seeing stars," start over from the beginning, to make her cum again.

Women are fun like that. But, again, some may not want or need or have time for "Yes, sir, could I please have another," as Charles Dickens' legendary character little "Oliver Twist" eternally begs.

Or, move face to face with her and kiss her on her lips, letting her taste her juicy love wine from your loving and gentle mouth; which, again, will say a lot about how much she's into it with you or is into her sex is naughty or cleanliness issues or anti-whatever-she-thinks-and-feels, if she says "now" to her own taste, but expects you to bathe in it and drink it like fine champagne.

Or vice versa, when it's your turn to taste "cream kisses."

But, now, with her all AGLOW from your lovemaking, it just may be:

- your turn to receive oral,
- the right time to make full loving intercourse, in whatever positions and types you two may do together,
- or just the right time to curl up and **really** "sleep together."

"I wiggled…"

"…against the desperate feelings running up my spine and twisting round in my belly and below, but he held me fast, sucking on me, on the secret me, tasting me, as I bucked against his face without control."

"His tongue flicked here and there, then skewered me, right into me, making my pussy run with tart juice, and teaching me a million new things about my own . . . swollen, begging need, while he slid one long, thick finger inside slippery me."

—"Laila's First Cunnilingus" from *Neale Sourna's North Coast Academies' Diary*, Volume 1 Number 1 [NCADv1n1]; available now, ebook and/or print

----

NOW, BACK TO YOUR DELICIOUS MAIN COURSE

RE-WARNING: Don't plan it the same....

Never think of cunnilingus as boring or sidetracking foreplay that leads to the MAIN EVENT.

Cunnilingus IS the main event for her, and it can be wonderful event for you, too.

In fact, think of it more as a delicious course, like food, not as an event. A huge Thanksgiving turkey dinner is great, with its many courses and constant nibbling, but so is a single, delicious, cream-filled Twinkie®, when you're hungry for one.

Don't plan it or play it the same every time; sometimes you have a little C time, sometimes a little "F" time with a penis or appliance or fingers).

Back to School, for Your "ABCs"!

A **lot** of people swear by this one.

But, you shouldn't be swearing, you should be swirling. Place the tip of your tongue to the left or right of her clitoris. Now, use your tongue like a writing quill to write your alphabet "A-B-C."

Your tongue's movement as you "write" with your tongue quill will send a thrill of lovely sensations throughout your lover's lovely body, as your "writing" gives just the right amount of contact to both the clitoral hood and her clitoral head hiding beneath it; unless you're one of those who bears down so hard you rip through the paper.

No ripping, okay?

This also it gives **you** something **specific** to focus on, instead of overfocusing on, "Am I doing this right? Does she love this...?" Etcetera.

Which takes all the fun out of giving fun.

For this fun little practice, you should also be creative.

Okay, **breathe**. Creative isn't **that** hard.

Try this, for instance, instead of spelling A-B-C, you can also spell out her name or words such as "I Love You".

Of course, you can write **other** letters of the alphabet or brief words, like "love," **in any language.**

Learn how to draw the character "love," in Chinese **(there must be one)**, or just draw a heart, with an arrow through it!

Game: A-B-C Sex.

You can also play a simple game, by asking her to guess what words you're spelling **before** she reaches her orgasm!

But, don't be surprised if she hasn't a fucking clue. And don't get mad.

It's a game.

A sex game.

A fun sex game.

And you're communicating.

Remember, I said that was **really** important? It still is. It ALWAYS is.

Sex, Sexual, Loving, Creativity.

Sexual loving loves creativity.

Think of it, feel it in your body and heart.

Don't just think of sex and loving and lovemaking as "technique," you're making love, or at least **having and giving really great sex**.

So, there are a **lot** of variations that you can do with your flexible, sensitive tongue, to keep your partner guessing and on the edge of explosive, moaning orgasms you lead her to.

* * * *

The speed of your tongue-writing also plays a very important part for her; try luscious slow, try tickly fast, try something in between or a bit of both. She'll let you know which she loves or if she wants them all, and in what order.

And, if she doesn't, remind her that communication goes both ways, you can't make her feel REALLY good, if she keeps the details of what does feel good to herself.

And listen and watch and look for those cues, in her body and breathing and sounds, if your lady is still too shy to let out a solid little birdlike "peep."

And never forget to kiss her, here and there, every now and then.

Begin slowly, **always**.

Or, it'll seem like you're rushing her, and forcing her to reach her peak, in from 0 to 60 in a few seconds or minutes flat. Not good.

Slowly. Always.

Only increase your speed, after you **know** she's significantly and most definitely aroused. When she "has a need for speed."

Women's Advice: " 'Alphabet Letters' is Absurd."

"Ron Jeremy, the legendary porn star, says some women love it clockwise, some like it anticlockwise, some like an up/down stroke, and, well, yada-yada-yada.

"Meaning that you don't really need to actually write out alphabet letters with the tip of your tongue; except that it gives you a process that'll slow you down, and not rush for results.

[Sex is a process, not an end all be all goal.—NS]

"Merely try various tongue and lip motions and then let her tell/show you what works.

"Try:

- Circle around her clit.
- Direct pressure right on her clit.
- Leisurely licking up and down.
- Holding your tongue still, but moving your head instead.
- Fast little snake flicks of the tongue.

"Try it all and see what has the best effect **for her.**

"I mean, okay, if it really helps you to 'spell out the letters of the alphabet,' in order to understand what action best inspires your woman to cum, then, so be it.

"But the real point is that when you find a motion that works well ... STICK WITH IT!

"Because, when you reach letter 'S' and the poor girl is suddenly bucking her crouch against your face—DON'T CONTINUE on to fucking letters 'T,' then 'U,' and then 'V.'"

For god's sake, lover. Stick with slippery 'S.' Oh, yessss!"

Clitoris Circling.

Gently place your soft tongue to one side of her clit; then use your tongue's tip to make slow, circles around that area.

Remember: **always** begin with slow motions, to warm her up to the feel and to intensify what she's feeling from you—**think lazy circles, perhaps a figure eight every now and then**—then, increase the speed little by little.

Think of the slow motions—.

No.

FEEL the slow motion for your tongue and lips upon her in the same way it feels when she slowly moves her soft hair against your lips, cheek, arm, or whatever body part.

It FEELS soooo sensual, doesn't it?

But it doesn't, does it, if she **whips** you with her hair?

That can come later, by the way, when you're ... when **she's** all whipped up from **all your slow mo action driving her need** for **more from you.**

Only when you see, hear, and feel that she's nearing her orgasm(s), and about to cum—**she may even tell you**—add a little more pressure, then a little more and more; going **faster and faster, around and around** her clit area, letting her need build—.

Until milady POPS!

Clitoris Sucking.

Gently suck on her soft clitoris, softly sucking it into between your soft lips, then let go. Like you do in the summer with the top, sides, and bottom of a melting and delicious Popsicle®.

Be gentle, as you begin, stay away from biting or using your teeth, and even **be careful of pinching and nipping with your lips**, without testing with her.

Ask.

"Do you like this?"

If yes, continue, if she says no, **don't** do it again, not until she asks.

"Can I try something?"

Only if she says, "Yes," continue, and if she likes it continue more; but, again, if she says, "No," or says, "Yes," to your experiment, and then anything disapproving like, "What the hell are you doing?" or "Stop it."

Then, do as she commands, STOP. And go back to where you left off, and she loved it, then go on from there, with another creative, loving, pleasing approach.

As you suck on her clit—**you're not a mechanical vacuum cleaner, so don't suck her fillings out the hard way**—slowly increase the intensity of your attentions, as you see, hear, and feel that she's getting hotter and more turned on by what you're doing.

Warning: Highly aroused.

*This skill method is recommended for **when she's highly aroused**, because suction too early, for many women, can put too much painful pressure on her intimate clitoral area too soon; bringing everything you're doing to a screeching halt.*

A woman's clit is much like a man's dick in that way; it needs to be engorged, before you can do any heavy or aggressive handling.

Women's Advice: "Stop Heading Down on Her…"

"…like a pussy-heat-seeking missile."

"For lots of guys, maybe even **someone** you know well, nothing's as exciting as having a woman you're into start touching your package or begin unzipping your fly, to head down south, as early on as possible in a make-out session.

"Because it feels good to you, and mostly because it takes away any insecurity and uncertainty about whether she will or won't; because that way you definitely know she's into you, too, or at least horny as hell, and you'll probably get some more, as well, besides the head.

"This is NOT—**I repeat**—NOT the case for nearly all women. And probably 99% of the women you'll get with.

"If you go STRAIGHT for her genitals or even start tonguing her mouth immediately after just starting to kiss, in most cases, it'll NOT be like in the movies, which are pressed for box office time.

"It'll NOT make her feel **great** and **hot**, because she's actually not turned on enough, yet.

"And, unlike it is for you, it WON'T chase away her uncertainties and insecurities, by seeming to confirm that you're all that into her.

"A woman's usually pretty certain already that you want to sex her up, and she'll be in various stages of deciding about whether she wants to actually have sex, with you."

* * * *

I read long ago in "Glamour Magazine" that when women are often planning to have sex with a guy, it's a decision she's made within the first half hour, or even first ten (10) minutes, of meeting her man! **[It may even have been less, but I can't seem to find the reference.]**

But... then the guy does a turn off, and she does a mental/emotional turnaround. No sale, dude.

* * * *

"What will quickly make it win or lose for you, generally, is how ready you are to **show her** that **you're fully into her** and **her sexual needs**; not just scoring new wet pussy or easing your own randy itch.

"So, diving instantly for her pussy, while clothed or the first time you're both naked together, if ever, is completely **not** the golden path of demonstrating to her that you're sensitive and responsive to **her** emotional and physical urges and needs.

"If she believes for one moment that you're just trying to get laid, and not digging **her**, in particular, well, for most women, **that's a serious buzz kill**.

"And you're not coming **[or cumming]** back from that, bub.

"So, okay, it's like this. The majority of women, who orgasm, have to get worked up a LOT, to get to that proverbial "fevered pitch," when there's **no friggin' way she'll say no to anything**; especially wedging you between her luscious thighs, NOW!

"So, unless you know your girl partner is seriously into quickies, when you dive straight for pussy, you're cutting your throat, if you think you have even the slightest significant chance you'll ever see her lovely, wet and all-hot-for-just-you genitalia.

"Which means you'll NEVER get her off.

"Bye-bye.

"It's easy, it's proactive, it's fun; spend time getting to know her and her body, don't think of it as just stimulate her, kiss, stroke, lick, caress and now can we DO IT?

"SLOW completely DOWN. You're making love, making a playmate, perhaps a repeat playmate, not in a race, guy. So, again, get to know her and her body, EVERY INCH OF HER, by:

- slowly and actually feeling for yourself and her, the joy of slowly and sensuously kissing her body's flesh, where it's chilled, or warm;
- licking, because she tastes good, and make certain she can tell by your reaction that she really does taste good, not just you saying so; and
- caressing and truly feeling the texture of her skin, its hair, its gooseflesh, and every other part of her body first.

"Do all this, until she's so worked up, and pushing against your face and pulling you to her. Then, there's no way, no doubt that she's wants you.

"Now. Down where it counts. NOW!

"This is no shit.

SexSinger: Cunnilingus

"Because when she's gotten a worked up by you, don't underrate the power of your lips and your tongue and your gentle fingertips teasing and tantalizing **[to build up sexual tension, but not give its release, yet]**.

"And the power of your lips, tongue, and fingertips to touch, to kiss, or to lick her most sensitive areas outside and around her pussy; especially her sensitive inner thighs, seldom touched lower stomach and abdomen, and of course her magnificent mons pubis.

"You want to tantalize her and start her thinking and then obsessing about **when** you'll give it to her, get her there.

"BUT, not JUST yet.

"The power of creative suggestion to the mind; especially the sexual mind, is a great and potent influence.

"But, do eventually give her what she wants and craves, from you."

Oyster Practice.

Get a fresh oyster—**If you can stand to lick a raw slider, and aren't allergic!**—and practice.

The shell is the outer vulva and the oyster meat inner labia.

And, if you're lucky, you'll find a pearl to practice on! And then give to her. Now, won't it be fun watching her face as you tell her, how you got that pearl for her?

And, even if you don't find a pearl, get one and tell her you found it that way, anyway. Or should have.

Either way, most women will get the hint and want a proving test run of your new lingual (tongue) skills.

Now.

"1-2-3 lift a pearl. 1-2-3 lick a pearl, or a clit."

And repeat.

You can also practice with fruit; a half slice of juicy orange, anyone? Work that tongue into each section, then flick and move around those firm little seeds. The next time it may be her clit.

Or gently trying to get to the tantalizing center of a sweat cream-filled Twinkie®. Ah, so much sweetness to scoop with your tongue tip and gentle suck out of its center.

===========================

"Dara sighed, which encouraged Tor, as he…"

"…stepped beyond his station and laid the Princess on her bed. He fixed his gaze upon her and felt his way along her incredible body, with his gentle tongue and lips, paying much attention to kissing and licking the lance scar on her upper, inner thigh, where the flesh is always most sensitive.…

"When he continued his journey up and down her, his long, thick black hair fell enticingly, purposefully across her, for he knew its power over a lover, by adding hundreds more 'fingertips' to the many sensations he generated deeply within her, making him pleased to see her now shiver as well, as he suckled her tongue, her lips, her chin, her throat, her ripe breasts, and her little cave of a navel, all of her soft, fragrant and tasty skin.

"Then he paused in the same place she had stopped with him.

"She seemed apparently overwhelmed by him, which pleased him exceedingly, because he wished to please her and because it distracted her from touching him too much.

"Her touches made him too urgent.

"He was between her legs, stalling at her dimpled waist and looked up at her, and smiled, knowing by the feel of her, the sound of her, that she wanted more of him. He slipped his fingers into her and she boldly writhed against them. He loved that she did not hide her desire or her pleasure from his eyes and ears, to leave him to guess, like so many others of her kind, of her status had before.

"She pushed him down her, as her urgent, wordless love sign, and he rolled his tunic and placed it under her firm buttocks, which, after he had his hands on their smooth, round promise, he had to remind himself he could not have all of her in one occasion.

"He did not have to remind himself that this teasing her, wooing her, was maddening while he postponed relieving the agony in his crotch, which was telling him he would not be able to bear not being inside her for much longer, as he gave her pleasure with knowledgeable tongue and long, well-educated fingers.

" 'Yes,' she moaned, and...."

— erotic novel work in progress "All Along the Watchtower, Book One" by Neale Sourna

----

BONUS GAMES.

Game: Hornblower.

Any of you who studied a wind or brass instrument, or who was a "band geek" can get vindication **with skills you already have**, and others have to learn.

Remember instrument "tonguing"?

Well, it's how instrumentalists, who play woodwinds like clarinets and flutes, or brass like French Horn, get those concussive, staccato, individually distinct musical effects, **without** using their fingers.

- "A short hair, like a tiny see. Hm, pube." Dry spit. "Ptuh!"

Game: Red Light, Green Light.

Yes, the old children's game is for adults, too.

Only let her control when and how long you lick her ("Green Light") and when you're still ("Red Light"). At a certain point, you may hear that all lights are all green all the way home!

Game: Feather Your Nest.

Invest in a fine, clean **(sterilized)** feather, one that has some firmness to it; perhaps one that has a firm top edge and soft sides, like goose or turkey.

Don't use the hard stem, scratchy end, you might cut or scratch her tender flesh.

Alternate licking her and feather tickling and stroking her with the feather, as you lap at the swelling contours of her secret flesh.

And, so, well, "Tonight She Comes (Cums)"—The Cars.

You can also try this little game with a soft fur object.

No. Not the family cat! Or its tail.

Try, perhaps, instead, a soft sable tipped—**Yes, its sable fur.**—artist's paintbrush; lusciously, delicious soft, and has all sorts of possibilities, and comes in many sizes.

And there's more, of course, that you can do together, or you for her.

Be inventive and create a few new variations of your own between the two of you; transforming boring, rote, loveless technique into creative, personal, and fresh lovemaking, SexSinging.

POSITION(S). GET A MOVE ON.

If you're just licking her vulval lips, over and over, and tickling over and over in the **same spot**, or in the exact **same**, unvaried way, she'll get used to it real soon and you'll make things boring pronto.

You can't climax from boring.

So, avoid turning exciting cunnilingus into a tedious, nonending routine of tongue lashing. However, varying your cunnilingus positions will help.

Remember, this is musical and harmonious; boring and tedious is bad for adults, unlike when you were ten you never tired of "99 Bottles of Beer on the Wall" or of "Row, Row, Your Boat"; but when anyone mentions THOSE songs to most sane and undrunk adults like us to sing, we cringe and whine, "Ahhhhhhh!"

So, sing Seal's "Kiss from a Rose" not "99—."

Hey, I was singing that!

"69" [Tell the Kids, "It's the Year the Mets Won Their First World Series!"]

One of the best positions for cunnilingus, and it won't give you a stiff neck, and whether you both can truly keep at each other the full time will depend on health, comfort, and the different timings of cumming.

However, if there's a choice here—**I take that back, WHEN the choice arrives**—help her cum first; most guys usually won't take as long to climax, as a most women.

And, besides, if this is a warmer for you for a full fuck; definitely take her there first, and then she'll be REALLY READY for **your** main event, AFTER **her** main event.

Just like a visual 6 and 9, turn around so that your legs are by her head and hers by yours. This allows both of you to enjoy your oral sex play at the same time, as cunnilingus meets fellation. Or cunnilingus meets cunnilingus.

"Sing out, Louise!"—Mama Rose, "Gypsy"

The one "bad" thing is that it's harder to concentrate on giving joy when you're receiving it at the same time.

"Try it, you might like it."

And, if not, mistakes are fun and sexy, too. Just stay relaxed and make certain everyone who needs to cum cums.

And don't bother trying to make it porn film sex, where both of you cum at the same time. It won't happen, and if it does, it probably will never happen again, or most likely won't, or, well, you get the idea.

It's a fiction ideal to sex up the mind, getting both body's at cum state, at EXACTLY the same time; especially, when you're enjoying receiving it so much you can barely focus or can't focus at all on giving.

This study, though, is about giving, so, you may have to let six cum then nine cums, or nine cums first and six gets to cum afterward.

You'll work it out, hm, fun it out.

Our goal is relaxed, happy, and fun real sex, and not "EXACTLY on time," stressed out stuff that will kill the mood nor is it about carnival porn tricks. Well, not unless you both really like that, then be my guest; but you newbies are warned.

Backward. More 69, Kind of.

Yeah, it's good ole "69" **[in French soixante-neuf (swah zahnt newf)]** again, almost.

It's actually just kind of "6" or just "9." This isn't BOTH of you "eating out" at the same time, like 69, this is taking the choice of helping her cum first.

Period.

Without all the distraction for her of trying to make you cum, too, and of you getting so caught up in your cumming you check out and steal the buzz from her and blow.

Her buzz is usually harder to get and keep and get to the top; especially if you add:

"Are the kids back, yet?"

"Is **that** your parents?" and other such distracting, sex buzz kill—.

"I forgot the wash; someone might steal it!"

So, no stopping cunnilingus for your handjob, or your blowjob, or your cock in her cunt, or in or between other parts intercourse, until your woman cums first.

Period.

It's just practical and sensible; because the happier and more relaxed she is the happier she can make you, right after. Happy girls don't bitch, or get headaches.

You'll get your eight minutes of blowjob; or so the pros say is all it takes, and that's being generous, if you've seen her naked and already have her on your mind.

Less, if it's cock fucking cunny, because cock loves cunny and was made for her.

But then, cock loves pretty much any hole, especially attached to a female; real in flesh or faux in plastic vinyl.

So, your legs are by her head, hers by yours, now get your head down in there, my friend, cause you're actually facing her vulva "downwards" or "backwards" to the position when normally kneeling for pussy prayer or lying flat on your belly between her knees.

Being "on her six **[o'clock]**," to paraphrase air pilot talk, naturally puts you into position for "downward" **(clit to vagina)** tongue lick strokes; instead of your usual vagina to clit licks.

Again, you must communicate between you, by words, signs, grunting sounds, sighs, or whatever, with your lady, as some women find the "normal" or "upward" tongue strokes on her clitoris uncomfortable, **extremely** uncomfortable, especially when they're not fully aroused enough.

This position—**so I'm told**—best combats and literally reverses "uncomfortable, **extremely** uncomfortable". Try it, and see if she likes it.

Doggy, or, as I prefer, "Doggy-Doggy."

Similar to "Doggy," during intercourse. You're both on all fours with you behind, with your head down to suck and lick her vulva dog to dog, or dog to bitch, so to speak.

Some feel this is "kinky." I am not some, but there you are.

Facesitter.

Yeah, that.

She deliciously squats over or on your gorgeous, willing face, giving her more control over the sex action, and you a view that is supreme.

However, the length of time your lady can kneel, squat, or sit over you or on you, provided you can hold her weight, while she **fully** sits comfortably and directly on or over you, depends entirely on how physically strong and/or rested you both are.

Don't do this if she has a heart or lung problems.

And be careful if she's considerably heavier than you, same for women with considerably heavier lovers, as anyone who's had a heavy heart attack victim collapse on them and completely pin them down; sometimes for days! And it made the news!

Doggy Sit ["I think I just made this one up!"]

This is a cross between Doggy-Doggy and Facesitting. She's on all fours and you lie between her legs, both heads in the same direction, and she, again, schmooshes her lovely parts down into your face.

She can schmoosh against you, and you can pull her to you, or elevate your head, with or without pillow; and she can rest on her elbows, like most men normally do while fucking in traditional Missionary Position.

[Tsk-Tsk, those sexually busy, sanctimonious, overly religious missionaries of old. Yes, the position is named after them by the Polynesians who thought the Mishies were boring and laughable, with their only one (1) sexual position.]

"Knees Up, Honey."

She lies on a flat surface with her feet flat but her knees up and you lie belly down with your head between her thighs; in reverse of Doggy Sit.

Most women like this arrangement, because it allows completely full access to their vulvas, and they can completely relax.

But, you, however, can get stiff necked pretty easily. So, try placing a pillow beneath her bottom to help raise her vulva to a more comfortable level for you, or perhaps a pillow under your chest or raise up on your elbows, or not, which ever is most comfy. You'll find it.

Legs Flat.

This is similar to the knees up position, except she leaves her legs flat.

Some women feel more in control in this position.

Both knees up and legs flat can be varied simply by moving yourself on or off the bed or table, and kneeling beside her. Just make certain it's comfortable for both of you, or used as a break in your movements around each other.

Knees, Fluid Movements, and Agony.

You can, with some of these positions, put one or both of her knees over your shoulder, for a change in position and access to her good stuff; whether lying flat, lying on your sides, standing, or kneeling.

There's a variant there, use a wall like a bed, so to speak. And try it standing or she's on the table and you sitting, with her knees over your shoulders.

Whatever you two do keep your movements fluid and relaxed and easy. And remember that, even when it seems **she's not doing anything**, but just lying there flat on her back, lying still for too long can become agony.

Personally, lying on **my** back for too long kills me.

So, move it, both of you.

Or she'll have a shooting or excruciating cramping pain in her spine just when you've coached her to just about—.

"Ow!" And that's not a good **ow**. Relaxed, fun, and comfortable.

Keep her guessing, "What's next?" and thinking, "This is **so** great! And fun! When can we do it again?"

As you lead her to rippling, trembling, or exploding orgasms.

Variety, unpredictable, fresh. But keep it simple and **about her**. And keep your "nose to the grind," so to speak, for your best success.

============================

"Then his touch,…"

…and then his kiss, as he kissed and made love to every part of her he saw and touched; making her moan for the first time. Ever.

"Stop!" she cried. He stopped.

"Almah was panting, over warm and dizzy, with spots before her eyes, while yet lying flat and still. Well, trying to lie still, for his lovemaking maddened her long married, but yet virginal, untouched body to move of its own volition.

"She looked and Hoy was there, not angry, but attentive, eager, exceedingly attentive, as always.

"And her own attention realized that she felt the heat and presence of his fine body, yet missed him, missed his gentle touch, his soft kisses, his warm breath, his … love for her.

" 'Don't stop. Resume. Please?'

"He didn't speak only touched her, kissed her. Everywhere. Where she had and where she had never been kissed before.

"Her lips. Her face. Her neck. Her arms. Her hands. Her shoulders. Her breasts. And, oh, her breasts and belly and … below.

"Oh, below, she moaned in her mind, trying not to say such a thing aloud.

"She wantonly opened her legs wide to him, at his gentle coaxing, as he moved to lie between her trembling thighs.

"She wasn't certain what he might—.

" 'Oh!' No one, absolutely no one had ever kissed and licked and sucked upon her *there*. Or *there*, or....

" 'Oh, mon dieu! Please.' He wasn't certain if that meant 'Please, don't stop!' or 'Please, cease and desist!'

"He stopped.

"And in moments, as she gasped in speechless bereavement at the loss of his touch, her pelvis gently thrust its glorious splendor up to his face, mutely begging...."

—erotic novel work in progress "Annamarie Makes a Match" by Neale Sourna

---

The ONLY Sex for Some.

Oral sex is the ONLY sex for many couples, and as the **only** sexual, genital activity they do together, **finding a truly comfortable position is enormously important**; so is thoroughly enjoying it together.

The best positions, to some, are usually those in which the love receiver is in a dominant or "top" position, kneeling or lying over her partner, giving her the most independence, by choice of movement and control of intensity and access to her body.

But some others prefer the much more relaxed, and laid back "subordinant" position or "bottom."

Try them all.

Mix them and use them in different orders.

Be **uncomfortable** for a short while, for the excitement of it, then get comfy and REALLY get to it. Yum.

MORE on COMFY POSITIONS. Yes, MORE.

Again, she may want to kneel or squat, straddling your head, so she can lower her vulva down to you, by her own control.

What works best for the two of you together will largely depend on the **actual physical angle of her vulva,** which can vary between women, and of your mouth, and the level of comfort for you both between these to mouths.

Placing a pillow under your head can raise it up to the level of her vulva. Or placing a big soft pillow or a folded comforter or quilt beneath her hips and lower back, so she can rest her weight on it, while still keeping her pelvis elevated and available for you.

When doing longer, extended love sessions, it'll be completely too tiring and an actual physical danger for either of you to continuously support or hold up any substantially heavy part of either your own or your lovely partner's body weight; no matter how light she says she weighs, or how strong you say you are.

Don't forget the dining and kitchen table, if sturdy and well balanced are a good idea, and come with chairs made for **eating**.

Also you can try a clean kitchen counter—**no salmonella near her nether parts please.**

Or try an office desk, preferably one in a home office or one you know is absolutely secure from security camera views, or viewing from homes and offices, even on the 80th floor, in some cities.

You can make a comfy spot on the floor together, on your sides; with a futon or camping bags, pillows, or blankets, or Arabian Night carpeting.

Try lying at right angles to each other, forming a "T," with your head inserted between her legs, and resting on her inner thigh.

She may have to prop her topmost leg open with several pillows, rest it on you; depending on your actual angles of intersection, while you lie either in front or behind her.

The actual physical structure of her genitals and your comfort together will determine exactly what is possible.

So, contrary to an idiot I used to work with in an electronics store, and who should have kissed his cute wife's ass everyday for stooping so low on the evolutionary tree, or for being so low in self-esteem, or really actually truly in full spiritual love with him, and marrying personality-challenged and dumpy him, of all people; he **often** said, "All women, once you stand them on their heads, all look alike."

Yes, he said this, in public, and more than once, and to women in particular. **Maybe he thought he was being shocking with women he could never "have"?** Shocking being as close to a sexual coup as this kind of guy gets with the really hot and secure and undesperate ones.

Back to more lovely and loving people.

A woman with a clit that projects outward, and which is apparently "long," or "well-developed," her partner can actually suck on it, just like a little penis.

With a woman with a tiny or hidden clit, her lover may only be able to lick at it.

A woman with full, well-developed inner labia **(inner vulva lips)** may like to have them sucked.

While those with thin or absent inner labia from birth; or if removed by "female circumcision[32]" **[Female Genital Mutilation (FGM) Diagram 1 and See Endnotes for more].**

* * * *

---

[32] Female genital cutting (FGC), also as female genital mutilation (FGM), female circumcision or female genital mutilation/cutting (FGM/C), refers to "all procedures involving partial or total removal of the external female genitalia or other injury to the female genital organs, whether for cultural, religious, or other nontherapeutic reasons." *[See Endnotes for more and/or Wikipedia http://en.wikipedia.org/wiki/Female_genital_cutting]*

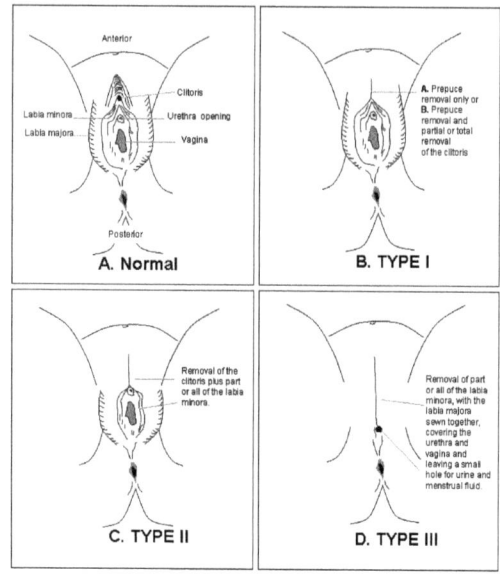

FGM Diagram 1:

Image shows average, uncircumcised **(natural)** female anatomy versus the different types of Female Genital Mutilation.
[http://en.wikipedia.org/wiki/File:FGC_Types.jpg] [33]

* * * *

And, depending on the type she's had, she may not like or possibly may be less likely, or even wholly encapable of or able to enjoy being sucked on.

Or even possibly enjoying any of what's been described throughout this book.

But, in this world economy, travel, and cross cultural marriage and love, one should note this.

Also, your ability to make love together this will always depend on her present anatomy **(physical and hormonal)**, her emotional ties with you, and your understanding care of her.

Make an appointment with her gynecologist for the both of you and find out what may or may not be possible.

But try anyway, if she's game, because doctors don't know everything. I've known them to say certain women will NEVER become pregnant, and their grown children would beg to differ.

Remember, she has an ENTIRE body to be made love to, so don't forget her inner thighs and more; some women can cum from attention to them as well.

WARNING: Don't break rhythm.

There is one important rule though, about her pleasure, unless you intend to tease her—and

---

33 Ibid.

aren't afraid she'll kick you in the head— keep up your rhythm and intensity, once you begin bringing her to orgasm. Absolutely nothing UPSETS A WOMAN more, during cunnilingus, than having her partner break their rhythm, or wander off THE spot, when he's on the verge of triggering her orgasm.

===========================

"I know, I could've just *taken* her, I..."

"...could've just *taken* her, I achingly wanted to; or one of us could take me manually, to take the edge off; I achingly wanted that too, but the self-inflicted, excruciating wait for her seemed right, particularly after what she'd just said about him. I'd seen his selfish impatience first hand and I didn't want to be like that, *like him*, with her.

"I wanted to wait for her, so to speak.

"I felt her relax against me; then started over, a little quicker this time, to get back to where I'd stopped. I put my lips and tongue to her natural fruit scented and flavored body and strove to delight her however I could, which plainly was a great deal.

"She'd been a bit tense before; evidently waiting for me to strip and hurriedly dive in like good ole Hopkins would've; without any joy in it for her. But, this was *my game*, and when I play it, the way I play it, nobody's better at it.

"*All modesty aside, of course.*

"Besides, a man's ... or a woman's rewards are greater, with a little patience and tender care. Especially, with the special ones...."

—*Benn* from Neale Sourna's "Hobble" *(a Year's Best Erotica Novel Award Winner)*; available now, ebook and/or print

----

MORE Warnings and Advice.

Women's Forum Advice: Again. "DO NOT Immediately Dive for Her Clitoris...

"...like a damned heat-seeking missile."

* * * *

It's much the way you feel, intruded upon when someone's dog, you've just met, immediately sticks its sniffing nose directly in your crotch, clothed, let alone **when you're naked!**

Yes. It's that bad, and that intrusive.

Or, it can make her feel put upon and stressed, in a like manner to how you'd feel or have felt when a woman is aggressively demanding sex of you NOW, and you're not into domination, so your boner's more "er" than bone.

* * * *

"Let your lady get warmed up and wound up, fully; because if a woman isn't sufficiently aroused, her clitoris will prove to be either **overly** sensitive or the flipside; **totally** insensitive, to **all** forms of stimulation; no matter how long you lick and hum and vibrate; until her boredom and soreness."

* * * *

She won't like it, you'll leave her unsatisfied, and you won't get invited back to her delicious oyster meal.

Wait for her hormones and lust level—**which vary with each woman, and from day to day**—to get flowing, and for her genitals to become engorged with blood.

Yes, **just** like a penis, the clitoris needs to be engorged and swollen fat for the sensational best results.

* * * *

"Make a slow and lengthy journey to her clitoris. Discover it, by 'accident.' She has **an entire body that needs attention**, not just her 'button.' And just like an elevator button, banging and banging on it won't get the results you want, not when **you** want it.

"So, take the long way around and down, by caressing, kissing, and licking her inner thighs and making love to other parts of her on your way around her full body wonderland tour.

"And when you do get in the vicinity of her sex, gently lick the joint, the area where her vulva and inner thighs come together.

"It's a lovely tease, and she'll love it!"

* * * *

Then work your way, no, PLAY your way along her body, with your warm breath on her here and there, lick a spot, then blow gently on it, also slowly kiss and lick her pubic mound and outer labia.

Women's Forum Advice: "Take Your Leisurely and Loving Time."

"Trace with your tongue's tip the length of the groove created by the meeting of her outer labial lips. Slip your tongue, by its tip and by its flat side **(front and back)**, along the dividing line of her inner and outer labia.

"If possible, gently draw her inner labia into your warm mouth and suck on them; this will gently draw blood into them; and NOT OUT.

"Don't draw and suck too hard, not unless she encourages you to do so, because she might bruise or bleed."

Editor's Note: It's not a great place for a Band-Aid®. Try one on your private fun parts.

Reminder: "Be Extremely Gentle."

Some women, no matter the age, only need a light touch; while others feel ticklish and will need a firmer but gentle touch. And still many others won't be able to stand direct stimulation on their clitoral glans.

SexSinger: Cunnilingus 61

Gently suck on her clit; to carefully draw blood into it.

Once finding a method of stimulation that's pleasurable to her, keep it up, sustain it, UNTIL SHE ORGASMS, if she desires one.

On occasion, she might not desire to go to climax, by choice or design of her body's varying hormone and emotional reactions.

If she's not able to experience orgasm, at present, or ever, continue your stimulation for as long as it's pleasurable for the both of you. It's really quite the same as kissing, and having a long session without climactic goal can be fun, too.

Cunnilingus needn't always or ever end in orgasm, because it's pleasurable to feel, and experience, and is a joy to share; and that, in itself, can be quite satisfying, too.

"This Pleasure's for Her; Watch, Listen, and Hear Her."

If she already knows what she likes, **listen and obey her instructions**.

If she's never had cunnilingus, or at least a **pleasurable** session of it, because it failed before, slow trial and error is required together.

Be patience; stay relaxed; make her laugh a little bit, to keep things loose.

Your tongue can get tired doing this, so be certain to also use your lips and tongue when you caress and suck upon her. Switch from kissing to licking to sucking to rest your muscles and not stop.

Extending your tongue full out, and it's not something most of us do a lot, so, your tongue can soon get tired. It's like going to the dentist, who wants your mouth open for like an hour; it can get tiring and hard to do.

You can practice and do exercises, or....

...get your mouth extremely close to her clit and labia. It is called "giving head," or "giving face," after all. And use short tongue strokes, with your tongue only slightly extended.

Insert Here. Maybe.

Some ladies NEVER love it, **but**....

Some enjoy it when your tongue's inserted into her vagina and you tongue fuck her. But, you may not be able to insert all that far, depending on the length of your tongue appendage; but, the most sensitive flesh of the vagina is near its entrance anyway, so she'll most always feel you.

Some also enjoy having a finger(s) inserted into her vagina, to stimulate her inside, including her G-spot, WHILE you kiss, lick, and suck on her clit.

And some love when your well-lubricated finger(s) are inserted into her anus and/or you just massage her anal opening, WHILE performing cunnilingus.

Also, once you've tried the basics and you've both gotten the hang of things, and love it, for variety, think of using dildos, vibrators **(many very discreet, even fingersized)**, and anal/butt plugs.

Some women really enjoy the expansive feeling of being stretched open or filled by you, WHILE she's being orally stimulated. And since you can't normally do cunnilingus and cock fuck, that's where busy, gentle fingers and loving, buzzing appliances come to play.

Literally.

Plus, a vibrator can make feminine orgasm more likely during cunnilingus, for some women, when it's otherwise impossible.

While the vibrator alone can result in orgasm, the combination of vibration AND YOU, being with her and helping her enjoy herself, can be even more pleasurable for her and result in a stronger, more far-reaching orgasm.

And don't forget the basic, most natural vibration, you humming against her, WHILE you're pressed against her secret parts. Yummmm.

==============================

"Leith's cunt was fresh and slick, as..."

...he fingered her and she wiggled.

"Ah!"

He parted her legs wide, pulled aside the fabric and looked at her softly haired sex. He glanced up, she was watching him look at her, and he slip his fingertips along her swollen, hot, wet flesh, while watching her reaction.

He parted the abundant and slick hairs then parted the swollen vulvar lips to her sex and glanced at her again watching him.

"Do you know what I'm going to do, young Leith?"

She shook her head "no." She was flushed with passion and life, her dark reddish brown hair spread out around her.

"Do you trust me to make it pleasurable?" A nod this time.

"Ask me to kiss you, Leith."

"Kiss me, Frederick."

He kissed softly upon her clit, an open mouth kiss with gentle lips ... and tongue.

"Oh, my."

"Leith?"

"Yes?"

"Ask me to make love to you."

"Oh, please, make love to me."

He licked the entire area of her sex, and she wiggled against the delightful feel. He pulled her closer, and....

—from erotic novel work in progress "Victoriana" by Neale Sourna

---

Male Advice

Paraplegic Man's Advice.

"As a paraplegic, I've a good method for cunnilingus I haven't seen discussed. We find that the best, comfortable position is her on her back, with her legs spread open, while I sit beside her waist, leaning over her hip, and putting my head between her thighs.

"She can thrust and move her hips, when she likes, as I keep contact with her vulva, and still not lose my rhythm.

"I can also insert one or two fingers into her vagina and tickle and pet her G spot, as I nurse on her clitty. And my other hand plays with her nipples and breasts.

"The perfect setup for us.

"Keep your same rhythm going with your mouth and both hands. It takes a little practice, like rubbing my head and patting my stomach, plus whistling too, but the effects on my her(s) are wild!

"They come quick; with powerful, multiple orgasms.

"I usually stop after about a half (1/2) hour to one (1) hour because their clit(s) become too sensitive from the use.

"Or, she has to catch her breath. LOL.

"I sometimes circle my finger inside, around her cervix, so deep inside, so not to overstimulate her **OMG-spot**."

Paraplegic Woman's Advice: "Braingasms."

"Did you know that people who have no feeling at all below the waist—people with spinal cord injuries, for example—can still have orgasms?

"It's true.

"My friend [edit], a paraplegic sex therapist [edit], has *physical sensations only* in her hands and arms, breasts (*one has less feeling than the other*), neck, and head.

"*Yet, when her clitoris is stimulated, she can have an orgasm.*

"*Where does she feel her orgasm to be located?*

"*Well, sometimes she orgasms in her nipples, sometimes inside her head.*

"She reports that there is a *distinct* difference between *nipple orgasms* and the ones inside her head, but that both are wonderful.

"She has even discovered that by changing positions during sex she can have *multiple orgasms.*

"[Her] experience illuminates *the presence of numerous previously undiscovered neural pathways by which orgasmic energy can travel through the body to the brain.*

"The more I study orgasm, the more convinced I am that *orgasm 'happens' primarily in the brain* and that *the intensely pleasurable feeling in our genitals*—the kind that usually accompanies most of our orgasms—*is only one of the many pleasures possible with orgasm."*[34]

— Urban Tantra

Lesbian Advice

Lesbian Forum Advice: "Put Your Nose to Her."

"Your nose!

"While playing and teasing her labia and vagina, with my tongue and lips; my nose tip is close to her clit.

"I gently rest it on her clitoris or move my entire head in a circular gesture, nose tip against her, while kissing and sucking her inner labia. My nose extends my stimulation coverage area!

"One lover had such an awfully sensitive clit; I could hardly touch her, without causing her pain. My own is more sensitive, sometimes, like during my menstrual period.

"A good tip I've learned, in giving oral pleasure, even with a sensitive clit, is to simply **RELAX my tongue**.

"Most people mistakenly stiffen their tongue, and licking her hypersensitive clit flesh with their hard tongue tip, just as oral sex begins.

"WRONG.

"Relax your tongue, instead, and take your time, lovingly licking her ENTIRE VULVA area with the soft flat of your tongue; and relaxing you tongue's tip to lick full out, like when licking an ice cream cone.

"Don't gouge with the tip of your tongue, since that can be painful, or even ticklish.

"Go smooth and flat.

"Then, test a few slightly firm licks, to see if she likes it, then play with a more firm or more soft tongue, depending on her instructions.

"Don't forget to lick the inside of her thighs and her pubic area, too.

"I often find that a woman with a really sensitive clit also needs more lovey-dovey loving, like holding and 'loving' love touches, BEFORE she can be sexual.

"If your lady feels completely loved and safe, BEFORE you get naked together, and BEFORE you get to her clit, her body will more likely respond better and more eagerly to your lovemaking.

"My wife orgasms come best, when I lie between her thighs, and lap at her in an upward motion. And I tongue her, too, in a soft building to firm swirling (circles or figure 8s) motion.

"It sends her out of this world, with multiple orgasms. And, it's great for me, a huge pleasure to bring pleasure to her, to the woman I love. There's nothing else like her joy for me."

---
34 Carrellas, Barbara. Urban Tantra. Softcover. Berkeley: Celestial Arts, 2007. Page 85.

Men's Forum Advice: Warning on Fingering.

"Some women **absolutely** DETEST having someone's fingers inserted inside them, and/or having their clits sucked.

"So, pay particularly intimate attention to her body language, and all the sounds and sighs she makes, that will indicate whether she is or she's NOT enjoying what you're doing.

"Pay attention to her giving impatient sighs or snorts or huffs of disgust, moving away from your face, or her breathing returning to its normal, everyday rhythm.

"Do experiment; with caution, and with respect."

* * * *

Experiment little by little, and if she gives you a direct **verbal**—like "No" or "Stop" or "What the hell?" or even if she gives you **nonverbal** directives, that sound like she's not into it...

Stop at once.

If there is a division, a question in your mind of what **her specific meaning** is, because it seems it can lean to either side...

Stop at once.

Don't let yourself feel or ever say to her anything like: "You're clueless, and don't even know what you like."

Which may be somewhat true, but still, she knows what feels better to her body and her emotions and is comfortable to her mind, much, much better than you ever will.

Just like you know better how it feels to get kicked in YOUR genitals.

No matter how much she's "suppressing" or "ignoring" or whatever **you believe** is going on in her, let it go. It's hers to deal with. You're here to help her know herself and enjoy herself better, not boss her around or think and feel for her.

So, be easygoing.

If her behavior bothers you so much, that you can't leave it be, maybe you should consider moving on, or give her just a little more time, to understand herself and communicate what she needs to you; as soon as she figures it out.

[Editor's Note:

And it may just be that the woman you love and want to give the ecstatic gift of cunnilingus to may NEVER be truly comfortable with it.

So, again, don't chide and belittle or whine her to death about her feelings or inexperience or whatever, since lots of lovers, who're willing to muff munch for hours, are terrified and go all anally tight themselves, when having someone diving to intimately lick around or stuff something deep into THEIR orifices.]

* * * *

"And, flipping all of this around, some eager women LOVE to have their clits sucked or licked hard, and harder, or pulled and pinched a bit with your lips.

"But DON'T try this not unless she constantly says 'harder' or 'more' or some such indicator, while you're loving her. Do what she says, until the lady tells you to stop.

"You also may want to try to suck and lick at the same time, while you also moan. I've been told that my moaning makes 'delightful' vibrations!"

* * * *

Or give her pierced clit ring a tiny bit of tug! But, check first, don't assume ANYTHING. Or mistakenly rip anything! Ouch.

"Orgasm: After Injury *(Physical, Emotional, or Spiritual)*."

"...Injury survivors can experience orgasm and this ability is not strongly related to the level or completeness of injury. Some of us, for that matter, find sex even better than before injury.

"There is growing evidence that sexual knowledge, sexual self-esteem, and time since injury are related to the ability to experience sexual pleasure and orgasm. It seems that knowledge is power, power fuels self-esteem, and self-esteem opens the door to sexual pleasure.

"Orgasmic sex requires turning in to our sensations—IN the MOMENT—and forgetting about *[imperfections, fluids, body scents, etc.]* and making embarrassing sounds.

"It means not worrying about performing up to some *imagined standard*. And it means forgetting what we learned in the past about what is and isn't pleasurable *[in THIS MOMENT]*."

—*The Ultimate Guide to Sex and Disability* [35]

More Forum Advice

Women's Advice: "Any oral is great oral." NO. It's Not.

"Keep in mind that, unlike with most men, just being willing to "go down" on her and begin licking all about doesn't mean she'll come, no matter how you do it.

"Women's orgasms while with another person are a highly emotional AND extremely intimate, physical thing.

"So, if you can't get both her busy mind and unfocused senses fully focused for eager and willing pleasure, she won't get off."

---

[35] Kaufman MD, Miriam, Cory Silverberg M.Ed, and Fran Odette MSW. The Ultimate Guide to Sex and Disability. San Francisco: Cleis, 2003. (Kaufman, Silverberg, and Odette p. 57)

[Editor's Note: Even if you lick and kiss and suck her raw all day, or night.]

Women's Advice: "Listen! Take notice!"

"Some women aren't the least bit shy about saying what they want you to do or about exactly what they like, which keeps you from having to guess, especially when making love to her is new; like on your Wedding Night together!

"But, many women will be TOO embarrassed to bluntly or even obliquely convey anything useful to you, by word or gesture, about themselves, while having sex.

"Either way, whether she yaks it up or barely answers "uh-huh" to your questions; **listen carefully** and **be highly attentive** to ANY noises, sounds, and movements she makes."

[Editor's Note: Quivering with smiling delight is great, and a yes, making tight, tense twitches with disapproving sounds, isn't, that's no.]

"If while you've got your head buried 'down there' you hear something—**an ecstatic intake of breath, a moan, a 'yes,' or if she begins to buck against your tongue and face, in a slightly less than controlled way**—continue what you're doing, you're on the path to glory.

"But, if she quiets down, what you're doing's not working, at least, **not anymore, if it did before**. Humans get tired of the same stroke; **like singing your one and only same song, over and over again.**

"Move on to another spot or try something completely new, until she begins responding positively again. Then, stick with this new action, until she comes or wants you to do something else.

"Also, if you hear 'No,' 'Not there,' or 'Ouch!' NEVER go back to that move."

[Editor's Note: Not unless she's into pain and instructs you to do so. And that's a big if, usually. Don't assume; you could end up in court for damages and criminal intent against her nether parts. No. I'm not joking. Otherwise, have fun.]

"Do realize that many women are a lot more sensitive than other women you've known, in her private area. So, even though your last partner **loved** having her clit nibbled, **don't assume another one will love it, too.**"

* * * *

If you do, you may get a heel to the schnoz.

However, if she says, "Right **there!**", "I'm **almost** there!", "I'm going to cum!", or "Don't stop!"

* * * *

"Well, DON'T STOP.

"Keep doing what you're doing, and hold on, as she thrashes about, and bucks on your face like a bronco!

"Just keep up your consistency.

"There is NOTHING worse than being about to peak, and your lippy partner decides to break for a minute, change his tongue motion, or stop completely and ask for a damn blowjob.

"There's a special hell for people like that.

"Once her momentum's broken, it can take a long while, a long, LONG while, to get her back up there again. Or she may NEVER get there, again, for that time.

"So, unless you and your partner are into denial and teasing, lick it till she's screaming in ecstasy, and thanks you when she's done."

Women's Advice: Communicate. Ask for "Tips."

"Never think or feel that asking her how she likes to be touched or given pleasure implies that you're clueless about what you're doing. It, in fact shows that you DO know something, that you don't know EVERYTHING ABOUT HER, and DO care about her wellbeing.

"While you're just getting to know her, or even long after you've known her well, never be afraid to ask her, 'How's that? Do you like that?'

"Let's face it, some days you feel like lemon pie, the next chocolate cake. And, so it is with lovemaking. There's nothing more boring than the same Ding Dong® EVERY time.

"I love it. It's so sexy to hear my partner ask, even when he knows me well, because I know he wants ME to **feel really fantastic,** and that my feelings for something he does might occasionally change from time to time, through no fault of his, or mine, even."

[Editor's Note: Our human bodies are complicated, with billions of nerve endings, and hormone combinations, triggered by emotions, concerns, and health.]

Game: Her Slave.

If you're favorite girl's just a **little** less shy, tell her you're going to be her "slave" for the evening, or, at least, at her complete command, like in the "Red Light Green Light Game," if slavery makes her nervous.

Tell her you're there for her, and at her full beck and call, with your only personal goal being to encourage and help her to have pleasure, and that she needs to tell you, must tell you, or point to EXACTLY what you need to do to and for her.

When to do it; and how to do it.

When to stop and to go.

Or to be given the command to "Please me," until she says: "Stop," "Go," "More," or any other such wonderfully interesting thing.

And throw in a few heartfelt "Yes, my mistress," which just might please her, and help her get turned on enough, to hand you the essential key to how to make her feel delighted.

But, if she's able to, ask her to SHOW you, directly, and actually demonstrate to you what exactly gets her going and off. She doesn't have to complete it, but show you how and where to touch her.

Fast?

Slow?

Hard?

Soft?

Vibrations?

Slow vibe or fast vibe?

You can even ask her to masturbate, so can watch her, which'll be exciting and binding for both of you.

You can even masturbate at the same time, so she won't feel completely on the spot, alone. And when she's looking fully turned on, and about to cum, focus on her, and make certain she sees your interest.

Ask to take over her stroke, but don't wrestle it from her, if she's too far gone to stop; just take notes, and once she's caught her breath, ask to give her stroke a try.

And throw in a hearty and loving, "Thank you for showing me your pleasure, my mistress!"

And ask if you may kiss her or show your enthusiastic, loving thanks in some other fashion she desires.

But, really, depending on how you say, "Thank you, Mistress," it could make her giggle and relax, and feel sexy and powerful, too.

Game: "Sweet Nothings" and "Puppet."

But many, not all, women, depending cultural attitudes and ethnic background and her own personality, will simply be far too modest and too embarrassed to do something as open and bold as any of this, or just fully intimidated by the whole concept.

So, try this alternative. It might make her feel safer, and less trampy, slutty, etcetera.

Stand, sit, or lie behind her, spooned against her; so she can feel you, but not see you face to face. Nuzzle her, touch and stroke her whole body, and whisper "sweet nothings" in her ear, and get her all "bothered" and "turned on."

Don't forget her back, across her shoulders, and neck, down her spine to her lovely ass **(outer bits, save the inner for when she's REALLY warmed up)**, the backs of her legs, all the way down to her feet.

Worship ALL of her, and then she'll KNOW you're not "Just after ONE thing." If she lets you muss her hair, then you KNOW she's there with you.

Now, you can do all of this before a mirror, or not. It depends on your girl.

A blindfold for her might be nice, too.

Or just one for you.

Or, perhaps, a blindfold on both of you!

Then, give her "full control" over your hand, like a puppet, her very own living marionette, and that **she should masturbate herself by using and guiding your hand, just as if your hand were her own.**

Think about it, YOUR HAND is her new sex toy, that'll she'll teach to obey her and give her, her very next orgasm.

The best about this is that your shy girl won't have to see you directly watching her, as she explores, teaches, plays, and cums.

It's simply hot, intimate, and a lot less confrontational, than words or fact to face lovemaking, or face in crotch, as you warm her up to more adventures.

[Editor's Note: And a variation on this is to place a mirror or few so you both can see what she's doing and you both can see each other, indirectly. Some shy girls, modest girls really love that. And, don't forget the blindfold variations!]

Another big plus is that you'll get to see **exactly** how she normally touches herself, which means that the next time you go down on her, you can do exactly the same thing, but with your lips and tongue.

Or discover a very close variant, in case she's like "Secretary" **(2002, film)** and lies on her tummy, with her hand between bed and her, while she finger masturbates, for the extra pressure on her clit.

I'm sure you'll figure out something that'll compensate and please her.

Right?

My hand's to my ear, I'm listening. What've you got in mind, for your loving her?

============================

"Ladies of the English Harem"

" 'He said I should have the Ladies of the Harem attend my needs. What does that mean?'

"There must be some mischief about it, she felt, as with most things with these people, but the anticipation buoyed her curiosity, as the Ladies, lead by the motherly Migs sisters bathed her and washed her long, wavy black hair, and dried her and anointed her, and then altogether bedded her.

"There was a woman upon every part of her, it seemed.

"And they'd trade places and trade places and Alora came and came again; and opened her eyes yet swimming with distant stars to gaze upon he himself, newly returned, standing near her bed, watching her, as the Female Harem attended her needs.

"Without thought, Alora loved his gaze upon her naked lushness, as she came again, *because* of his heated gaze, because of the many hands and mouths upon her, and because of the new maid Rhia, whose mouth was already highly educated on how to pleasure a countess.

"Without thought, on his part, he slipped out of his clothes and with both physical and silent command scattered the Ladies of Harem, who drifted away like silk on a breeze, except Rhia, who yet hungrily licked and sucked and drank her lady's sweet juices, which could not cease, not in his presence, until he grabbed her by her red hair and pulled her away and took her place of feasting.

"Alora closed her brown thighs around his dark head and pushed against his exquisite mouth, with no more thought of harems, when she had the master of all stables and harems fucking her with his facile tongue, holding her squirming against his face, as she grabbed his black hair and came in a great many shudders and thrills."

—from erotic novel work in progress "Silver Blood" by Neale Sourna

----

SexSinger BONUS: Add Fingersex.

Begin your lovemaking with simple exploration of her, y'know, going where no finger—**of yours, anyway**—has gone before. On or in her.

Only start with fingers, as you'll have better control over them, and a better sense of when they're touching the wrong thing, and exactly how deep they are.

Save all your toy objects for after you've gotten better acquainted, and more familiar with each other in sex.

Just like a baby, fingers and toes first, toys later.

Try a varying number of fingers, but do start with one, to see if she even likes being probed.

Never forget her lips and mouth, her chin, the sworls of her sensitive ears. Kiss her and touch her with lips and your fingertips, and let her become accustomed to you doing so, and slowly work your way to where you hope you're going.

Backtrack a little. No. You're not losing ground. She's not ground.

It's a game, with a little touch of mystery.

She'll get an idea of **where** you're probably going to, but she doesn't have to know EXACTLY when; and—.

"Watch out, that alien's got an ANAL PROBE!"—as paraphrased from "The Simpsons."

No hurrying, right?

Smile, relax, and be lovingly sensitive. And so will she, in answer to your smile and sensitivity.

Your attitude will give her more trust and CONFIDENCE IN YOU than all your words of, "Trust me," or my personal fave, that ALWAYS sets off mental alarms, "I won't hurt you."

"What! Who said 'hurt'? There's going to be pain? What're you doing?

Wha—?" **I think you get my crazed, tensed out drift.**

Poking around "down there" is always a loaded matter, since most women only have tampons or their gyno's tortuous, cold speculum devices and medically, uncomfortable probing fingers in their most private area.

Which is as about as lovely an experience as most men feel when being felt up by their urologist and his big, long proby fingers. At least a male's doctor doesn't stick metal up his ass.

Be gentle, go slow and be kind, as you explore and probe and finger massage different parts of her, like her vulva, her clit, her vagina.

Don't jab your hand into her and bruise her with your hard knuckles, and don't forget earlier to cut and file smooth your nails.

No spontaneity here. Be clean, trimmed, and filed. No icky guck under your nails, giving her an infection. No jagged nails scratching her most sensitive and intimate skin.

And, later, if you do go the toy or object path, be kind to her cunt, be inventive; but no sharp, breakable, or spiky objects.

Not unless she's asked you to, and you also agree, as well. Lovemaking is a mutual affair, and NEVER one-sided—**if both of you are conscious, and you should be**—one person gives and one person receives, always. Sometimes you both give and receive at the same time, but that can become one-sided as soon as one comes closer and closer than the other to cumming's culmination.

No "Performance." No "Task." More Training Your Senses.

Think fingerfucking, WHILE DOING ORAL; but, let's back up, again, just a bit; to go over a few finer points of nonverbal communication and bodily sensitivity.

Remember our Sensuality Game? Click back through the Table of Contents, if you need to. Then come back to here. I'll wait.

Hi. Welcome back.

Remember to take your time, and use ALL of your senses.

Look and truly **see** her texture and her changes; because when you do this, you'll enjoy it more and because she will enjoy you enjoying her, which will take her far beyond the "Does my butt look big?", "You don't really like how my armpits, crotch, whatever smells like?", and the like. Love her and show her you love her, and she'll love you back.

I'm not talking "all encompassing love" here, maybe, but not necessarily, just "Geez, Terry's really into me, I like that, I LOVE that, guess I'll hang with Terry a little longer."

That kind of love.

Feel with your fingertips, with the backs of your fingers, with the palms of your hands, with your cheeks, with your lips....

Do listen because, if it's quiet enough in your love grotto, sex cave, the sound of your touching her may be there for you to hear, as well, as your touch moves over the fabric of her clothes or the fabric of her skin, or hair.

Always take in how **you** feel and how **your** senses feel while interacting with her, with her skin against your skin, **feel how your <u>entire</u> being focuses more and more on just what your fingertips touch, or doesn't, hasn't touched yet, and also how you feel. Outside and in.**

Also don't forget the simple joy of smelling her hair and her skin, before you get to "the good stuff."

And smell her other hair—**if she has pubes**—and her sexual, sensual skin when you have gotten to "the good stuff." But, then again, ALL OF HER IS **GREAT** STUFF!

Remember also, that your senses, when properly focused completely on the two of you and how you FEEL together, will put you both in the same erotic place and mood faster and deeper than any words.

============================

"I *loved* him touching me. He…"

"…slipped his long, thick fingers along my slit, parting my soft curls of pubic hair. I loved watching him see me, all naked and all for him.

"My sex flesh was swollen, sweaty, and musky as a wild thing in heat.

"I wanted, needed him to touch me more.

"I lifted my knees higher and wider, without him asking; disgracing my ballet teacher, but opening me, displaying myself to him. 'Just like a wanton slut,' is what I'd heard an old woman say once, like it was a bad thing."

—Laila from *Neale Sourna's North Coast Academies' Diary,* Volume 1 Number 1 [NCADv1n1]; available now, ebook and/or print.

BEST OF BOTH—MULTITASKING: Clit AND G-spot!

Putting Your Finger(s) In.

Get her warmed up, and wound up; but not tense.

You know what to do. Love her, love her all over.

Kiss and lick and suck her inner thighs, and her labia and clit especially, to get her nice and slick wet with her natural, hot pussy juice; but only, if she's not **already** slick and hot for you from all your loving attention to all the other fine love zones of her delicious body.

Enhance the entire experience for you both, constantly, but especially for her, by continually kissing, licking, and sucking her vulva **(inner and outer lips)** and clitoris throughout.

For best dexterity, sense of feel, and subtle control, use your writing hand, and its first two fingers **(one if she's tight, and especially only one, if she's** still a cock in cunt intercourse "virgin").

Use your fingers closest to your thumb **(your Jupiter or pointer/index finger and your Saturn or middle finger, y'know THAT finger, the one you flip people off with).**

Now, either wet them with your mouth, or hers, or—**preferably**—with her cunt juice; whichever turns you both on the most and has the wettest slickness. Her own juices should be more "oily"/slick than saliva, but then you've been kissing and loving her all over, haven't you?

Tell me you didn't skip straight to finger in?

Of course you didn't, you want her to have a GREAT time with you.

Anyway, your lady should be quite slick wet for this to properly work. If it's necessary for her, especially for medical reasons, you can also use a fine water-based "personal lubricant," and an edible one. You can find them at your local drugstore, online, and at great loving couples store all over.

WARNING 1: Nails.

Make certain YOUR NAILS ARE TRIMMED and FILED SMOOTH, without LOOSE or RAGGED BITS, and NO SHARP edges.

Tender flesh ahead.

WARNING 2: No wet spot.

If you didn't lay a towel or nice soft and absorbent blanket or robe beneath her before, for the oral, do so now, to save your sheets for dry sleeping afterward, your couch for wet-stainless sitting, or your best table from wet damage.

Cool, huh? You're both gonna love this.

Slide one finger into her cunt, gently into her vaginal entrance, starting with just one, to see how she likes the feel of you inside her, feel how wet and slick she is, or isn't, and because if she's tight, you'll have to gently work up to more fingers.

Slide in with the print pad of your finger facing the same way as her face and belly button, with your nail towards her spine.

Slide it in firmly, but slowly, and gently, as far as your finger(s) will go, without definite resistance, and not with too much pressure, or force.

So, don't poke her or slam you finger in to the hard knuckles.

If she is extremely tight, or there is a lot of wetness, but interior physical resistance still, start with one finger, but don't force it in her, tease and taste her some more.

The more she relaxes with you, and the more she's aroused, the more her vaginal muscles will ALLOW you entry.

Do note that a few women also have rather tight muscles here or inflexible hymens[36], which may obstruct entry or have DENSE hymens, see the film "Kinsey," and may need surgery to help in sexual entry.

Or to undo previous surgery, if her culture required her "sealed" at puberty.

No, I'm not making this up, if you skipped over stuff earlier that explained some of this.

Don't skip, she's important to you, isn't she?

And her enjoyment, as well?

Once inside her, tease her inner walls with your finger pads, and get to know her, and how she feels, and reacts to you, which will make her even more wet and "juicy," as the back of naughty girls' pants used to say.

When you feel she's ready for orgasm, and could use your help to get off and cum with more intensity, move your fingertips to her G-spot.

You've been getting to know her inside—**How she feels and how she likes you "feeling her up."**—so, you've probably already touched on it.

And yes, it's real and every woman has one. I still hear some say it doesn't which means, they've never "touched a lady,©" like the fellow asked in the Monty Python skit, "How does it feel?©"

Your lady's G-spot is a patch about 1-2 inches deep, and up, along her front wall, just past the entrance to her vagina.

Technically, it's behind her clit, but inside, on her FRONT INNER WALL. So, in, up, and more towards the entrance, than towards her cervix deep inside.

Do **not** poke her cervix**[; that's the inner, back "wall," at the top of her vagina, from where her period and babies come from, and sperm goes in]**.

"Ow!"

She will hate you for harshly poking her there.

Poke yourself in the eye, it's a similar pain.

Not really, but it'll make her laugh, probably.

The pain is probably more like having your nut sack pinched hard.

"Ow!"

You should feel, on her inner wall, a roughish or corrugated-feeling patch on that upper side; it'll feel rougher than the rest of her smooth muscled, inner cunt.

Make a gentle "come here," or "come hither" for you old school types, motion with your fingertip(s), by tenderly sliding and then gently rubbing your pads across that spot. Only press lightly, to tease and excite it.

It's much like when you're sliding your fingertip over the fingerpad of your

---

36 The hymen is a fold of mucous membrane surrounding or partially covering the external vaginal or opening of SOME women or girls, and forms part of the vulva, or external genitalia. A slang term for hymen is "cherry," as in "losing one's cherry" or "popping her cherry," *[as in the Jewish wedding ceremony, I believe, when the napkin covered glass is violently STOMPED on]* meaning losing one's *[her alleged]* virginity [to her husband], or lack of sexual inactivity.

laptop's fingerpad. Gently, she has priceless equipment. But you can vary the pressure and the lengths of your fingerstrokes.

You want to make her feel good. Not bang her into pain from the inside. I'm not encouraging or suggesting that in the least.

NEVER scratch or poke at her G-spot, it's quite sensitive, just use a flat fingered rubbing, like one does to feel powder like sugar on one's fingertips.

Hold her legs apart with your other hand, or shoulder, if you have to. You can even use your head or knees or whatever, depending on what position you're in, to hold her legs open, but **make certain she stays relatively still, or she might get hurt**, you may poke her wrongly if she's moving too much.

Squirming and Breathing Heavily. Her, Not You!

As you, with sexual musical delicacy, lightly press, slide, and/or gently tap your fingertips against her G-spot, she should start getting even wetter; with cunt juice, not piss. Unless you did poke, as requested not to, which just might cause her to piss on you.

More on this later.

If you're fingering and touching **(slight tapping, stroking in lines or circles, etc.)** her correctly, and she's happy with it, you'll hear a squelching, or wet sponge sounds coming from where you're touching her.

Keep sliding your fingerpads, over and over the area, and rhythmically keep time, a little tapping drumming, or you can even hum a song, your "our song?" to keep you on rhythm, or with the same kind of paced rhythm you might would strike up while sliding your cock in and out of her wet cunt.

Which will be familiar to her body's memory, if she normally gets off on that.

As she gets wetter and enjoys herself more, press more firmly, but never hard. The more she wiggles against the feel, the more firmly and faster you can do it.

Even when "banging" your fingers in and out, keep up an upward firmness, without poking or scraping, or actually slamming your knuckled fist against her. You don't want to give her a "black eye," or in this case, I guess it would be a black clit, vulva, and vagina.

Unless you want to get punched in your genitals, too, or she specifically asks that you do so, and signs a contract for proof for the law, later, when you argue about, don't be anything less than gentlemanly and gentle, mon.

Through all of this, she should be squelching, dripping wet, squirming and wiggling and OBVIOUSLY loving it.

If she's not, you should stop.

If she's says something like, "It's okay," or something else that sounds lukewarm or like she's just going along to please you—**which is not what this is about**—we're pleasing her, stop.

If she says it hurts, especially if she's said it more than once, STOP.

Contrary to what our various overlapping cultures have secretly and obviously filled us with, sex for a woman shouldn't be painful.

Be sure she's ALWAYS wet, and rewet with a fine genital, "personal" lube, if she's not, because ANY dryness will hurt her and bring your playtime to a screeching, painful halt.

This is lovemaking, not painmaking. That's another book, from another person.

Now here's the crucial part. When she gets close to ejaculation, she may say she needs to pee.

============================

"Ejaculation. The Joy of 'Squirting'."

"For women who live with incontinence, ejaculation *(which often results from stimulation of the G-spot)* may cause some distress. When women ejaculate, it looks, feels, and sometimes even smells a little like urine. [edit]

"Many manage to work through their initial fear *(usually with a few peeing moments along the way)* and discover that it is not the end of the world and does not have to 'destroy the moment.' [edit]

"If we have only negative associations about fluid involuntarily coming out of our bodies, it may be hard to experience what some women call the 'joy of squirting.'

"On the other hand, knowing that ejaculation is possible gives an opportunity to think in a whole new way about getting all wet during sex. If there is the possibility of shooting some fluid during sex *(whether pee or ejaculation)*, it's happening because we were in the throes of pleasure—which is surely a good thing."

—*The Ultimate Guide to Sex and Disability* [37]

If she has ANY concerns, or you do, just lay down a nice, thick, cushiony towel or two, or a thick, fluffy, absorbent blanket, or two—**have a sweet, good-hearted giggle about it**—and then forget about it; and let what happens happen.

Her clenching to not pee, on herself and on you, will keep her from relaxing and cumming. And cumming is a GREAT PLEASURE you don't want her to miss out on.

Women can inadvertently crap and pee while having babies, anyway, so why put so much stress on it now?

Prepare for a possible mess.

Relax and enjoy each other.

And have fun.

---

[37] Kaufman MD, Miriam, Cory Silverberg M.Ed, and Fran Odette MSW. The Ultimate Guide to Sex and Disability. San Francisco: Cleis, 2003. (Kaufman, Silverberg, and Odette p. 55)

"I Have to Pee."

She doesn't actually have to pee, provided, of course, that she did pee **before** you started; which she should've done, to alleviate any mental concerns or actual urinary pressure of feeling a need to pee.

Not unless, of course, that kind of pressure is her kind of fun.

Despite what she thinks she feels, and she thinks that because the spot you're touching is **right** near her bladder, it's merely a brief, upsetting sensation, that'll pass; but, you have to make certain she knows that she'll feel it in advance, or she'll be completely convinced she's about to piss all over your hand and face.

And you wouldn't like that?

Or would you?

KEEP GOING.

In fact, when she feels a need to pee, start doing it more firmly, because her orgasm is usually just about to cum.

About 10-50 seconds **[I didn't time this, someone else swears it]** after her pee sensation begins, she'll start to cum.

Now, in case you forgot, my multitasking friend, this is about cunnilingus, and this fingering gig is a bonus.

So, as you fingerfuck her, keep your mouth or put your mouth back to giving her cunnilingual joy, AT THE SAME TIME.

Do it to please and this woman will completely fall in love with your joymaking.

WARNING: Forbidden Pleasure.

Just so you know, and this is documented in some of the reference books used here, you may find some women, and your woman's not alone in this, will feel that this pleasure is UNBEARABLE and INTOLERABLE and will completely nix it.

Not because it feels bad, but because it FEELS SOOO GOOD, and she's been told, and taught, and beating down by culture, family, church and state that a WOMAN SHOULD <u>NEVER</u> ENJOY SEX, ONLY MEN DO. Women who enjoy sex and experience orgasms are bad women, amateur sluts, and professional prostitutes.

You may have to work a while to coax her out of this, or even get psychiatric/psychological help, too.

ANOTHER BONUS: Female Ejaculation.

When she starts cumming, as you give her cunnilingus and/or fingerfuck her, DON'T STOP!

Finger her more and more firmly, gently pressuring upwards on her lovely G-spot the whole time.

Some women will, some won't, but she could start to squirt or ejaculate.

SexSinger: Cunnilingus

She'll shoot transparently clear, sometimes odorless liquid all over. You did put down a towel or other absorbent material, right? There could be a lot, soaking you and the sheets, so be prepared.

Oh, and there could be joyful screaming and writhing, but it depends on the gal.

A certain blog/forum guy, who shall remain nameless, and who has given notes, swears that in his experience, as many as at least 97% of women are capable of having ejaculatory orgasms.

But his is not an official, organized study, my friend; as he alluded to all women but wasn't actually specific, and so I assume he meant the ones he knew in a biblical sense overlain in his mind to mean all women.

So take his advice and personal stats from above the above paragraph with a grain of salt.

Much like some who can't quite be trusted with their bowling scores; not saying he's wrong, but it is a less than formal study.

WARNING: Salt.

She's not a margarita drink, don't sprinkle salt on her and lick it off her tender parts. Salt scratches, a lot.

Hey, I've lived a rather sheltered life, and don't know everything, I trust in others' experiences to help me in mine.

Mr. Nameless also says that once your lady quirts she can squirt again, in one to ten minutes, depending on the lady and how quickly you get her back through her sexual peaks and valleys, but that you'll also have to press harder on her G-spot.

It's not a race, so don't race and hurry and push her to do it over and over to prove you can make her cum. She's not a hand puppet, so get over yourself.

Also for her to ejaculate in great volumes, have her drink lots of water and juice before you begin, to stay well hydrated. But not liquor and wine because the alcohol dehydrates and she won't enjoy herself as much if she's drunk, no matter what the romance and porn lit and the films say.

*Her getting high on the sex with you will reach higher and lasts longer, **without** the alcohol or other controlled and uncontrolled substances.*

One man's personally kept, and uncorroborated, stat record was seven, meaning that the woman he was with squirted seven (7) times, within forty-five (45) minutes, and then she passed out for six (6) hours, after they'd finished.

Whoo! Wouldn't that scare the Hell out of you, though?

Warning: Doctor's office.

Oh, do note that you may want to be subtle about the water or juice until you both get the complete hang of this.

Why?

Because women are often ordered to gulp down mass quantities of water, when at their g-y-n doctor's office. So, it may have clinical associations, which may, or may not, seem sexy to her. Depends on the gal if that's her or your combined fantasy...?

Her ejaculating is exhausting, physically, and dehydrating, as well, so be very careful, and check about her general health before enjoying such physically strenuous exertions, especially if you both try more than twice at one lovemaking session.

Also, in the basics, if you do your fingerfucking wrong, and poke and jab her too hard, and don't cut and file your nails in respectful pre-preparations **(like you were supposed to, kind lovers get more love, people)** or if she's on her period, she might bleed.

Her being on her period itself is usually okay, outside of AIDS/HIV concerns, in which case wear a condom over your finger or wear latex gloves.

Just make certain you don't hurt her, and stop immediately, if she's shrieking with pain, rather than pleasure.

You should always have a safe word with your partner, just because it's the sane thing to do and clears up any confusions, such as "Her 'no' means 'yes,' " and "Her 'don't' and 'stop' mean go," etcetera.

And you should **always** make certain she knows what you intend to do, AND double check that she's **always** fine with your proposed actions. And again, that your actual action is truly pleasurable.

I know it sounds exhausting, asking all these questions, constantly, but it's not.

It's communication and if you do it with the combined tones of loving concern and flirty playfulness in your voice, it'll be all cool.

No, you don't have to give her a written or verbal long list, by rote memory, but do use your words, like:

"Do you like that?"

"How's this?"

"I have a little surprise; tell me if you like it."

Hey, if you do something wrong, and have to stop it, you can always kiss her on her body at the spot or on her lovely lips, after each one, because one always get a kiss after a boo-boo, right?

============================

Focused Awareness.

...Two techniques you used in ... *focused awareness* (also called *attention*) and *imagination*. The use of the two of them led to *sensation*. [And] it can also help you increase sensation. Now try this little trick on your clit. Or your cock.

(Or for some of you, both!)

SexSinger: Cunnilingus

The technique of using your mind to focus awareness [*and imagination*] and move energy through the body is incredibly powerful, and it's not limited to what *you* feel; it also applies to what you can do with another person.

My lover was lying on her back. I was leaning over between her legs, tonguing her clit. She was enjoying it. I was busy writing the letters of the alphabet on her clit with my tongue.

I began to visualize sexual energy traveling up her spine, over her head, down the front of her body to her clit, and up her back and around again. **I was wrapping her in a kind of erotic egg of energy.**

She reacted almost instantly! Suddenly she began to moan and writhe, and just as suddenly, she was about to come.

I had very deliberating not changed anything I was doing with my tongue and my hands had never moved.

What *would happen if I stopped the visualization?* I wondered.

Again, I did not change anything I was doing to her clit nor did I move my hands. But I stopped visualizing the circuit of energy I had been wrapping around her.

Her energy fell like a stone. I resumed my energy circle.

Zoom — back to moaning and writhing. I stopped again; her energy fell.

The experiment over, I [silently] tongued, "Y-o-u c-a-n c-o-m-e n-o-w," on her clit, and she did.[38]

—*Urban Tantra*

"Go Forth, and Influence Women."

This certainly isn't the **last, final** word in cunnilingus; strive for but **don't expect** it to be "perfect," every time.

Because that causes unneeded stress.

And strive to make her feel wonderful and exceptional but **don't truly expect** to GIVE her HER ORGASMS.

Not to seem a downer, this late in the game, but we don't actually **give** her anything, we can only **encourage**, and she **accepts** it or doesn't or can't or won't.

Her body must cooperate, along with her mind and spirit. And heart.

She could be stuck with the kids on her mind or her hormones are just screwing with her. Or her heart, for whatever reason, is just not into it right now.

There's a secret about enjoyment: If your heart's not into it, the rest of you isn't either.

Try watching an hysterically funny movie when you're terribly sick, you won't laugh, not as much as you would if you'd been healthy and fully into getting

---

38 Carrellas, Barbara. Urban Tantra. Softcover. Berkeley: Celestial Arts, 2007. Page 30.

your laugh on.

So, be patient, with her getting her enjoyment on and with yourself helping her get there.

If it persists, and she's trying and willing, but nothing is still just not happening; go with her to a good doctor, who can check out her hormones and make certain that even though she's seems wholly healthy her hormone mix may be off center—**an alarming number of women fall into this category, especially with childbearing and menopause in the mix.**

You and she may need help from a psychologist, too.

But, first, give her some basic, easy help away from her worries and concerns. Do your dishes, put your kids to bed, pay and mail off all the bills, and she'll probably relax a LOT.

When we were kids, we alternated doing the dishes, but when adults it usually falls to only one of us ALL THE TIME, that's not relaxing or fun.

And let her SEE how much unconditional LOVE and OPEN GRATITUDE you have for her in particular, and for being able to "give," to encourage her pleasures and ecstasies, and the fantastically GREAT HONOR that is yours every time she has allows YOU to be THE ONE to do so.

So, go forth, and be successful with ease, my now wisely skillful buddies, and win friends and influence women, make them ecstatically happy with YOUR bliss-giving, SexSinging skills.

Make appreciative women sing of your importance to them and of your praises, in lovemaking with loving approval, and never say, "No," again, not to you, my glorious SexSinger.

—Neale Sourna

www.Neale-Sourna.com
www.SexSinger.com
www.PIE-Percept.com

Endnotes

[excerpted from Wikipedia January 2009]

Female genital cutting (FGC), also as **female genital mutilation (FGM), female circumcision or female genital mutilation/cutting (FGM/C),** refers to *"all procedures involving partial or total removal of the external female genitalia or other injury to the female genital organs, whether for cultural, religious, or other nontherapeutic reasons."*

Almost exclusively used to describe tradition, cultural, and religious procedures in which parents must give consent, because of the subject's minor age, rather than procedures done with self-consent. FGC is practiced throughout the world, with the practice concentrated most heavily in Africa.

Amnesty International estimates that over 130 million women worldwide have been affected by some form of FGM, with over 2 million procedures being performed every year.

FGM is mainly practiced in African countries. It is common in a geographical band which stretches from Senegal, West Africa to Ethiopia, East coast, as well as from Egypt in the north to Tanzania in the south.

It is also practiced by some groups in the Arabian Peninsula.

The country where FGM is most prevalent is Egypt, followed by Sudan, Ethiopia, and Mali. Egypt recently passed a law banning FGM.

A Greek papyrus from 163 BC. mentions girls in Egypt undergoing circumcision and it is widely accepted to have originated in Egypt and the Nile valley at the time of the Pharaohs.

Evidence from mummies show both Type I and Type III FGC.

The earliest evidence of male circumcision is also from Ancient Egypt. *[Approximately 2000s BC, predating the Moses claim around 1300s BC.]*

FGC advocates have claimed *the practice more beautiful, more clean, and cures females of a myriad of psychological diseases including depression, hysteria, insanity and kleptomania.*

FGC is often used as a means of control over "female virtue"; being a means of "preservation" and "proof of virginity," and is regarded in many societies as a prerequisite for honorable marriage.

Type III FGC is often used in such societies and the husband will sometimes slice his bride's scar tissue open after marriage, to allow for sexual intercourse for him.

Heavy stigma lies on men who marry an uncircumcised woman.

Women with genital surgeries are often considered to have higher status and value, than those without; including being entitled to positions of religious, political and cultural power.

Removal of the clitoris is often cited as a means of *discouraging promiscuity*, as it eliminates the motivating and physical interest factor of sexual pleasure.

Feminists and human rights activists disapprove of this practice because **it presupposes that women lack personal self control or the personal right to decide when and with whom they engage in sexual activity.**

The World Health Organization (WHO) uses the term Female Genital Mutilation, and classifies FGM into four major types (see Diagram 1), although there is some debate as to whether all common forms of FGM fit into these four categories, as well as issues with the reliability of reported data.

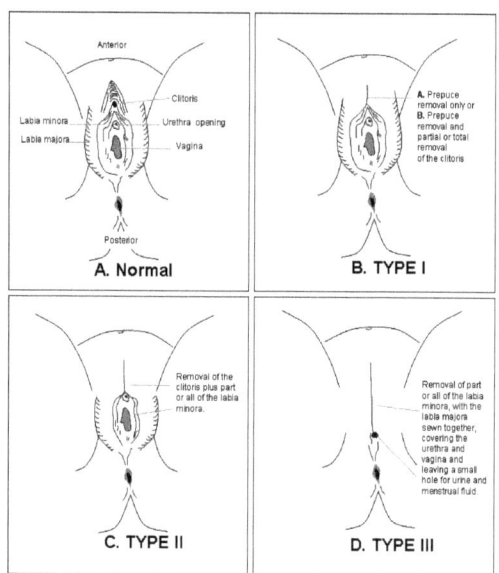

FGM Diagram 1:
This image shows the different types of FGM,
and how they differ to the uncircumcised female anatomy.
[http://en.wikipedia.org/wiki/File:FGC_Types.jpg]

Type I

The WHO defines Type I FGM as the partial or total removal of the clitoris (clitoridectomy) and/or the clitoral hood (prepuce) *[a slice of prepuce/foreskin is what is cut away in male circumcision, but not normally the penile head]*; see Diagram 1B.

When it is important to distinguish between the major variations of Type I mutilation, the following subdivisions are proposed:

Type Ia, removal of the clitoral hood or prepuce only;

Type Ib, removal of the clitoris with the prepuce. In the context of women who seek out labiaplasty, Stern opposes removal of the clitoral hood and points to potential scarring and nerve damage.

Type II

The WHO's definition of Type II FGM is "partial or total removal of the clitoris and the labia minora, with or without excision of the labia majora (excision)."

When it is important to distinguish between the major variations that have been documented, the following subdivisions are proposed:

Type IIa, removal of the labia minora only.

Type IIb, partial or total removal of the clitoris and the labia minora.

Type IIc, partial or total removal of the clitoris, the labia minora and the labia majora.

Note also that, in French, the term 'excision' is often used as a general term covering all types of female genital mutilation.

Type III: Infibulation with Excision (cutting away)

The WHO defines Type III FGM as narrowing of the vaginal orifice with creation of a covering seal by slicing and *repositioning* the labia minora and/or the labia majora, with or without the slicing away of the clitoris (infibulation)."

It is the most extensive form of FGM, and accounts for about 10% of all FGM procedures described from Africa.

Infibulation is also called "pharaonic *[Egyptian emperor/king]* circumcision."

In a study of infibulation in the Horn of Africa, Pieters observed that the procedure involves ex-tensive tissue removal of the external genitalia, including ALL of the inner labia minora and the inside of the labia majora. The labia majora are then held together using thorns or stitching.

In some cases the girl's legs are tied together for two to six weeks, to prevent her from moving, in order to allow the sealing together of the two sides of her vulva; leaving nothing except the flat wall of flesh from pubis to the anus, with the exception of an opening to allow urine and menstrual blood to pass through; see *Diagram 1D*.

[Editor's Note: Not unlike cutting off someone's lips and stitching them together

to fuse and seal together what is left, but leaving a small opening for small strawful of food and drink. Then, later slicing them apart, again, without a surgeon, when their marriage partner wants to tongue kiss, or let them throw up.]

Generally, someone perceived as having the necessary cutting skill carries out this surgical procedure, with only a local anesthetic.

However, when carried out "in the bush," this infibulation surgery is often done by an elderly matron/grandmother or midwife of the village, without anesthesia.

Wikipedia: **http://en.wikipedia.org/wiki/Female_genital_cutting**

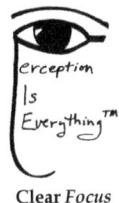

Clear *Focus*

PIE: P*erception* **Is E***verything*™
Clear *Focus*
12600 Rockside RD Box 192
Cleveland OH 44125 USA

www.PIE-PerceptionIsEverything.com
www.PIE-Percept.com
www.Neale-Sourna.com

www.ingramcontent.com/pod-product-compliance
Ingram Content Group UK Ltd.
Pitfield, Milton Keynes, MK11 3LW, UK
UKHW021321180426
11947UKWH00015B/1369